Aphrodisiac Adventures

Praise to Aphrodisiac Adventures

"Lillian Zeltser is a trustworthy guide on the natural stimulants trail, full of eagerness, passion, and respect for science, traditional wisdom and cultures. I support her mission to make these remedies and their uses better known in our culture and to raise public awareness of the impact our sexuality produces on every person's life."

Bruce Livett - Professor of Biochemistry and Molecular Biology

Aphrodisiac Adventures

THE KEYS TO USING AND UNDERSTANDING APHRODISIACS

LILLIAN ZELTSER

TM The Golden Seal image is a trademark and the slogan "To Health, Long Life & Pleasures "is the motto of Aphrodope Pty Ltd denoting a series of books, other publications and products relating to aphrodisiacs.

Publisher – Aphrodope Pty Ltd, Melbourne Australia

Series Consultant – Dr V.L. Zeltser

Editor Heather – Millar

Book cover design by Helen Christie

Photography by Evelyn Zeltser

Painted Illustrations by Christine Zavod

ISBN 978 – 0 – 6488046 - 0 - 4

EAN 9 780648 804604

Disclaimer
Most of the aphrodisiacs described in this book are unsuitable for people under the age of 18, those with ill health, and lactating or pregnant women. While most of the recipes in this book have been personally taste tested by the author, she does not take any responsibility for any reaction or impact on any individual. The information in this book is not medical advice or a prescription. It is based on the author's personal point of view and is intended for entertainment purposes only. Please consult a qualified healthcare practitioner before using any aphrodisiacs.

Acknowledgements

I am grateful to the many people who have helped me to write this book and to expand my vision to the true life's values throughout the years.

I especially wish to thank my husband, Dr. Victor Zeltser, who shared my obsession with aphrodisiacs for decades and greatly contributed to my knowledge of nutritional and herbal medicine and biochemistry.

Many thanks to Dr. Ivan Gulas, who believed in me enough to put this project together.

Thank you to many amazing people who generously shared knowledge, experience and wisdom of their ancestors to make this book possible.

Thank you to my friends who gave me a willing ear and emotional support during the years of my hunt for aphrodisiacs around the world.

Thanks to Christine Zavod, who artistically translated humble plants into hand-painted aphrodisiac illustrations.

Thanks to my daughter, Evelyn, who graciously spent time with me while I sat at the computer.

Contents

Foreword

"To Health, Long Life and Pleasures!" – Dr. V.L.Zeltser

Dear reader,

What would you think if I'll say that life without libido could be compared to eating a picture from a cookbook instead of a real food – it thrills and whets the appetite, but ultimately, doesn't satisfy?

Due to some fortunate circumstances which you will find in the next chapter, I discovered the power of aphrodisiacs early in life, which has given me many years to enjoy their magic and experience its delightful effects.

In over thirty years of being devoted to the study, practice and usage of aphrodisiacs, I have never met a person, who hasn't, either intuitively, openly or discreetly, been interested to find out aphrodisiacs they really exist – and whether they work.

The word 'aphrodisiac' tends to trigger people's immediate attention, as our sexuality had been preset by the nature to create most pleasant and intense feelings, which we are able to experience in our lives. However, the level of interest in the subject usually depends on a person's social, religious or personal attitude to sexuality, and their physical and mental limitations.

Regardless of nationality, gender, religion, skin colour or achievements, inevitably – sooner or later – the sexual drive of every single person on earth might declines due to either sickness or accidents, over-indulgence or extreme diets, medications like cholesterol-reducing pills (statins) or natural processes of ageing that are outside of our control. It had been proven that environmental or any other stress also contributes to the decline of sexual drive by increasing cortisol – the 'stress hormone' in our bodies, which reduces the production of hormones like testosterone, and neurotransmitters in the brain including serotonin and dopamine, which are responsible for our happiness.

However, the wicked human brain tends to preserve in detail those vivid, delightful memories of our sexual peak, which later in life can cause torment, making people long to experience those sharp feelings again at any cost.

Our sexual maturity awakens at approximately twelve to fourteen years of age and peaks at twenty-three to twenty-five. At that time, we experience feelings which are engraved in our memories as perhaps the best days of our lives. Thereafter, our libido is designed to gradually decline at the speed determined by many factors outside of our control; however this process can be reduced by taking care of its health.

Before we go any further, let's define 'libido'. In general terms, it is the ability of the human body to generate sexual energy, which enables us to feel excitement, and to fuel its acceleration into euphoric climax. In other words, libido is our sexual energy – driving force of our lives.

For centuries, we have been made to believe that the strength of our libido is directly related to our age, thus when it starts to decline many people tend to accept it and simply surrender to its loss. However, science and history prove that it doesn't have to be this way, as nature provided us with many remedies, which can maintain health of the most important thing we posses – sexuality.

My life-long research into aphrodisiacs and personal experience of them have helped me, my wife and many other people to maintain and preserve general health, sexual energy, avoid the traps of ageing, have happy relationships and continue to enjoy life's pleasures well into autumn years. I would like to share with you what I have learned about nature's gifts to humankind that are available to us, and to inspire you to take better care of your libido.

There is no one particular aphrodisiac that can work for everyone, as our bodies and minds considerably differ from each other. The only way to find the specific aphrodisiac, the one that will work for you, is through the trial and error of time-tested aphrodisiacs.

We are not talking here about strawberries, chocolate, champagne or oysters, or things that might send many people running – such as powdered rhinoceros horns, venom of scorpions, secretions of toads, sea slugs, human blood or other bizarre substances posing as aphrodisiacs. I am referring to proven ancient remedies, which have survived the test of time … and which I have personally experienced.

Identification of a suitable for you aphrodisiacs will largely depend on your physical, mental and emotional health, your common sense and determination, and ability to follow recipes.

The principle is simple – what doesn't appeal to your senses is not good for you! Trust your sight, touch, taste, hearing, sense of smell and pheromone receptors: they will guide you towards the most effective aphrodisiacs for you.

Please note that people with long-standing libido deprivation might not experience an immediate heightening of libido when they start this exploration, as their bodies may take some time to accrue necessary elements and compounds in order to 're-boot'.

This book is not a scientific work – it is based on the author's and my personal experementations with aphrodisiacs and life-long research of these hidden gifts of nature.

There are many scientific, medical and general works that have been written about aphrodisiacs – however, to my knowledge, this is the first book to focus on legendary aphrodisiacs and their specific effects, which can then be matched to each person's individual needs through an enjoyable process of experimentation.

Due to some fortunate circumstances which you will find in the next chapter, my wife and I discovered the power of aphrodisiacs early in our life, which has given us many years to enjoy their magic and experience its delightful effects.

Now, please embark on your guided aphrodisiac tour and dare to discover the power of aphrodisiacs!

- Dr. V.L.Zeltser

Introduction

The discovery of secret aphrodisiac formulae

Years ago I used to be ignorant and sceptical about the existence of aphrodisiacs until … one perfect, warm autumn morning in Paris…

The aroma of freshly brewed coffee mixed with the alluring smell of French patisseries wafted through the crispy urban air. I was standing at the counter of a small artisan café choosing something special from the menu that would please my husband's carnal senses. He sat with his newspaper at a tiny marble table, nestled in the shade of the old buildings on a narrow footpath opposite the Seine.

It was our wedding anniversary – 30th of October – and we were lucky enough to celebrate it in the city of love - Paris. Both of us had been born in the former USSR, where trips overseas were the privilege of Communist party leaders and celebrities, so the excitement of being free in the city of love was intoxicating for us.

Overwhelmed by the iconic views of Paris, the tantalising aromas of breakfast and our love for each other, we simply enjoyed the moment by cuddling in the soft autumn sunshine. The sounds of shop window shutters being thrown back cut through the still crispy morning air, signalling that the numerous old bookstores had been opened.

My gorgeous husband – a notorious bookworm – started to become agitated, even anxious as he planned to visit the many old bookstores snuggled there on the Left Bank. Since I do not share his passion for old books, we agreed to go our separate ways and meet up in a couple of hours at the same café.

While I walked through the labyrinth of historical nooks on the Left Bank, my husband conducted his dusty hunt for old treasures. His hard work was rewarded with the acquisition of two rare old books – a recipe book by the genius of traditional French cuisine - Auguste Escoffier, and *The Decameron* by Giovanni Boccaccio, a collection of erotic love stories written in the 14th century.

At the hotel, Victor was trying to mend the torn cover of *The Decameron* with sticky tape, when a folded page fell out of the book. I picked it up and read aloud the neat hand-written text written in Latin with the strange title - 'Aphrodope'. It looked almost like a recipe,

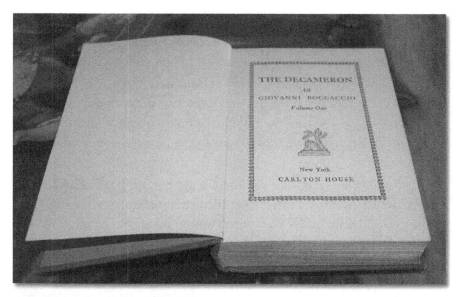

and although it didn't make much sense to me, my husband instantly recognised them as 'adaptogens' which he had researched under the direction of Professor and Doctor of Medical Sciences Israel Brekhman, while writing his thesis dedicated to the organic medicine of biologically active substances.

Mockingly Victor joked that 'Aphrodope' probably stood for 'Aphrodisiac Dope'and that it must be a love-potion recipe, purposely left in the book by the previous owner, who wanted it to be found by the next admirer of *The Decameron*. Then all of a sudden he proposed to test it out on our return home. Inspired by his optimism, I volunteered to help, not suspecting that this decision would totally change our lives.

Upon our return home, we tried to source botanicals listed in the recipe, however it was not such an easy task. After exhausting all local nurseries and herbal shops we decided to source them directly from their natural habitat – fresh and potent, where they synthsise to the maximum, their valuable bioactive elements. This decision delayed our preparation of the recipe for many years, since we were busy attending to the needs of our growing family and work.

Our very first trip confirmed that aphrodisiacs were not quite the gimmick we once thought. We discovered many effective aphrodisiacs and traditional aphrodisiac recipes, which were passed from one generation of native people to another.

The more time we spent on research and travel, the more my husband and I were sucked into the mysterious world of aphrodisiacs – and our interest in the subject was certainly fuelled by their unexpected efficacy!

We enjoyed learning about the part aphrodisiacs had played in certain historical events, mythical legends and folktales, the curious local recipes and their effect on us. Thus the hunt for aphrodisiacs became our life's obsession, which consumed most of our free time away from work and family.

Every holiday we travelled to a different place in the hope of finding new aphrodisiacs. After a while we realized that making the original recipe we had found in *The Decameron* was no longer our priority; we were totally captured by the actual process of finding new aphrodisiacs and discovering their powers.

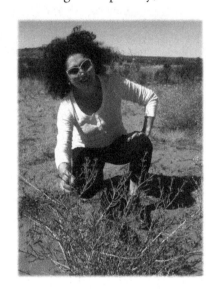

We had been lucky to meet so many brilliant scientists, amazing shamans, researchers, historians, sex therapists, cooks, herbalists, doctors, poets and native people, who shared with us their aphrodisiac experiences and knowledge. But most importantly we discovered that libido was commonly used around the world as a universal indicator of physical, mental or emotional state of health and aphrodisiacs as their fuel.

We threw ourselves wholeheartedly into research of proven aphrodisiacs, laboratory tests and travel, often entertaining guests at our special 'aphrodisiac dinner parties' with stories of some of the amazing experiences we had along the way.

Finally, after years of searching for the eighteen botanicals listed on the original 'Aphrodope' recipe, they had been collected. However, since it did not contain any instructions for preparation, it took several more years of trial and error for my husband to master an effective botanical extraction method, which could preserve their valuable bioactive components able to produce the required effect in living tissue or in a living organism.

In October 2009, after spending years and an absolute fortune on research, ingredients, lab tests, formulas and equipment, my husband managed to decode the remarkable life force of all 18 botanicals, and our hard work was crowned by a small test-batch of perfect bioactive aphrodisiac drink. It was perfect – potent, tasty, aromatic with the enticing deep red colour of aged Armagnac! My friends called it 'Love in a bottle'.

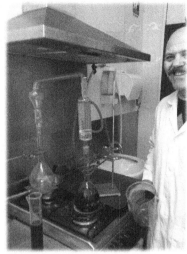

Most of that unique batch was used in tests and at the aphrodisiac dinner parties with our friends, who to our surprise kept on calling us back afterwards to ask for more of our love potion. To our joy, many of them confirmed experiencing extraordinary sexual rejuvenation and wanted more of it.

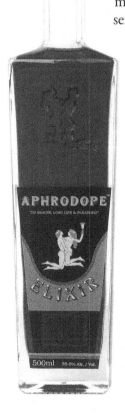

Realising the significance of our discovery, we decided to produce it commercially, and to avoid the hurdle of strenuous pharmaceutical inquisition, market it as a herbal liqueur – 'Aphrodope Elixir'.

Lastly, I would like to welcome you to the world of aphrodisiacs – the world of strong emotions, perpetual pleasures and healthy libido, which is supported by physical, emotional and mental balance!

I understand that this book is likely to be criticised and scrutinised by sceptics, as well as by the pharmaceutical companies and those who they feed. After all, who would buy their expensive, chemically produced medications if more people knew about humble and, often free of charge, natural aphrodisiacs, which have been proven to be efficient for over thousands of years?

13

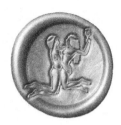

The Power of Aphrodisiacs

'The tragedy of a weakening libido is not in losing it, but in remembering how good it once felt having it!'
                                                                    - Lillian Zeltser

Like all living creatures on the earth, humans are sexual beings who gladly obey the rules of nature   – 'live and multiply!' – not only because they are destined to do so, but because of the powerful pleasure it gives them!

Why would anyone consider engaging in sex – or becoming parents for that matter – if not for the powerful physical and emotional pleasure that accompanies the sexual act! Researchers have found that regular sexual activity helps to raise the level of substances in your body that lengthen life span – such as DHEA, endorphins, growth hormone – and lower those that can shorten it, like high levels of adrenaline, cortisol and stress hormones.

People who enter relationship for reasons other than sexual attraction usually regret it later in life, as life without sexual pleasures, at any age, is wasteful and against all basic rules of nature. According to science, happy relationship, and feelings of love and sexual satisfaction increase levels of immunoglobulin – the antibodies, that play critical part of our immune response to bacteria or viruses.

There are many factors that can affect our sexuality,but luckely mother- nature provides many effective remedies, commonly known as aphrodisiacs, which are ready to help people combat these problems.

Unconciously, we are more attracted to sexually active people – they are usually confident, balanced and generally happy, and tend to choose our partners by their physical appearance. Those with signs of good inner health – like symmetrical facial features, strong bodies, long legs, blemish-free skin, white teeth, thick hair, straight posture, scupltured muscles – are considered to be attractive, as this signifies their ability to produce healthy offspring.

While wrinkles on the faces of sexually-charged people may attract partners, the signs of physical deteriation and low level of sexual energy indicate health problems, which intiutively repulse us. Unfortunately, rather than addressing their health problems, many people resort to cosmetic and plastic surgery, which can only ever mimic a sexy, healthy look, and cannot produce any real feelings of sexual desire or real satisfaction.

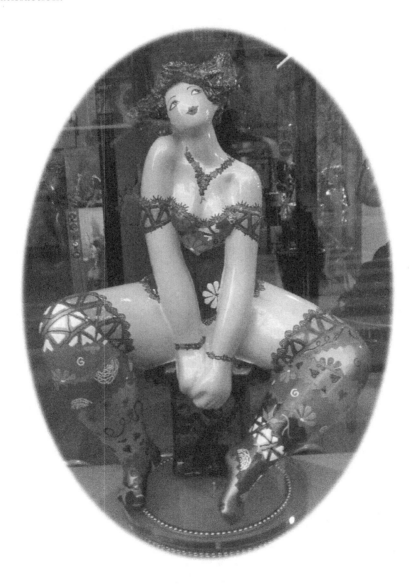

'You will never know the true value of aphrodisiacs, until your libido will become a memory.'   - Lillian Zeltser

While wealth or power can produce temporary euphoria, they are unable to compensate for a lack of sexual excitement controlled by our brain. After all, how many powerful and very rich people are there who are not able to experience real love, or build strong long-lasting relationships?

How many couples are bitter about their vanishing sexual attraction to each other, and how many couples blame their partners for their lack of libido instead of looking for ways to fix their problem? How many people really know about aphrodisiacs? Attract a life of happiness for your family by learning about the power of aphrodisiacs, create loving relationship, discover your true sexuality and start living your dreams.

'If only people knew more about aphrodisiacs' powers and learned to use them in everyday life, the world would be a better place!'
                                                          - Lillian Zeltser

As mentioned previously, there are many internal and external factors that can weaken libido, which subsequently may cause tensions between partners, especially those who don't talk to each other about their sexuality.

Often people are simply afraid of being misunderstood or judged, so they avoid talking about the issue or ask for help. They see it as a 'shameful' personal problem and often tend to hide the deterioration of their libido by blaming their partner for their relationship breakdown.

And yet, many of these situations could be avoided if people would recognise and use aphrodisiacs to restore and maintain their sex drive and emotional attachments, boundless sexual energy and limitless vitality.

Imagine how you'd feel if you would deliver the joy of truly feeling ALIVE for yourself and your loved ones?

'If people didn't enjoy sex, by now human kind would be long extinct!'
                                                          - Lillian Zeltser

Nature likes harmony and balance, and equipped both partners in order to enjoy their sexuality equally. However, due to some religious and cultural guidelines, which were based on socio-economical factors, rather than on the rules of nature, it has been – and still is believed in many counries that men like sex and need it more than women.

Thus, when men hear their partners excuses, such as headache or feeling tired, in order to avoid intimacy, they don't interpret it as an alarm bell - a cry for help. Instead, many see it as a personal rejection, which can lead a sexually unsatisfied partner to silent suffering, infidelity or search for another partner.

This wouldn't happen if people maintained an open mind towards sexuality and felt free to discuss it with their partner without fear of being judged. Nor would it happen if they learnt more about natural aphrodisiacs and their specific abilities, whether its to enhance, reboot or nourish their libido.

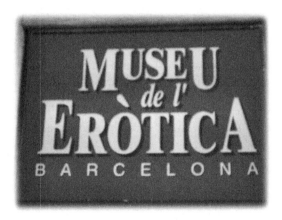

I highly recommended that you discuss your interest in aphrodisiacs with your partner, as a decision to explore this new world together will not only be more enjoyable, but it will be a bonding experience that can produce exhilarating results. It's fun to keep this little secret from the world and share your intimate experiences openly with each other, without fear of being misunderstood, discovered and ridiculed.

There is no magic behind aphrodisiacs! It is simply chemistry, physics and the process of evolution, where certain chemical elements, minerals

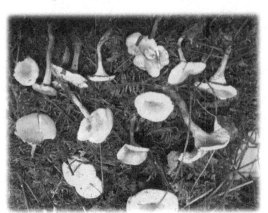

and other substances accumulate in order to enhance the chances of survival and reproduction of the particular plant or animal species. Those, who consume these substances might also be able to experience their power.

For thousands of years people experimented with

plants, animals and other natural resources, in hope that synthesised or accumulated in them minerals, chemicals and compounds that would promote the health of their libido. Fortunately for us, only effective aphrodisiacs survived the test of time.

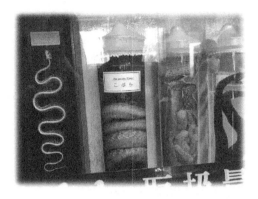

Take, for instance, pine pollen, which appears on the male cones of pine trees. It's erect, little tree-penises are loaded with phyto-testosterone destined to fertilise female pine cones with the aid of wind, insects or birds. European ancestors noticed that this light-coloured golden dust, fallen from the pine trees onto the ground, was sought after by animals in the spring heat. They correctly assumed it to be an aphrodisiac. So this is how they discovered its potency and ability to treat male version of menopause (andropause).

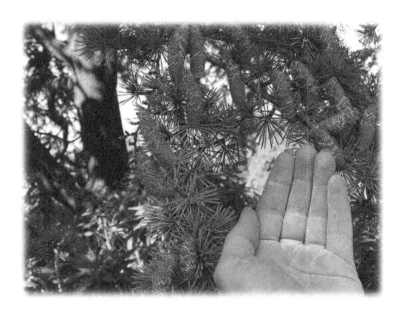

Chinese herbalists came up with their own effective version of the same remedy - Dragon Brew, which is made of ginseng, ginger, Indian mulberry, Mountain Flax seeds, horny goat weed and deer antler velvet. Remarkably, both remedies are still being used around the world today.

The best thing is that most of natural aphrodisiacs are free to take – they are around us! It's possible that instinctively you have been using some of these aphrodisiacs in foods or drinks, however you did not link your good mood or enjoyable feelings with the humble ingredient.

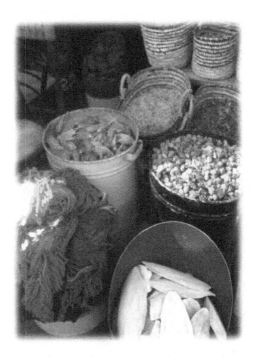

The exact level of your sexuality is known only to you and only you can take care of it properly. Since every person is different, you will need to experiment with as many aphrodisiacs as possible and in process, evaluate their effects. Through experimentations with as many aphrodisiacs as possible, in various different combinations, you will be able to identify your own personal ultimate aphrodisiac(s). In essence, the selection of aprohrodisiacs is very simple – what doesn't appeal to your senses is not good for you!

Likely, our senses are very powerful tools for guiding us towards things that can help us to preserve, maintain or re-activate our body's own mechanisms that support sexual drive. This explains intuitive changes of our tastes and habits, which are trying to direct us to the changes of lifestyle or substances necessary for our body to energize its mechanisms and keep us healthy. Every individual has their own specific needs and abilities to respond to these 'healing calls of nature', which control the health of our libido.

Whether you experiment with aphrodisiacs for reclaiming or establishing long-term sexual vigour through stimulation of glands and balancing levels of sex hormones and neurotransmitters, or want to experience a short-term burst of sexual desire, your body will recognise what works for you and reject what doesn't. Just trust your feelings.

So, unless you have health problems or abnormalities, listen to your own body and give it what it craves for – whether that's a certain aroma, herbs, caffeine, chocolate, fats, salt, erotic music, arousing incense, socialising, or simply cuddling or dancing.

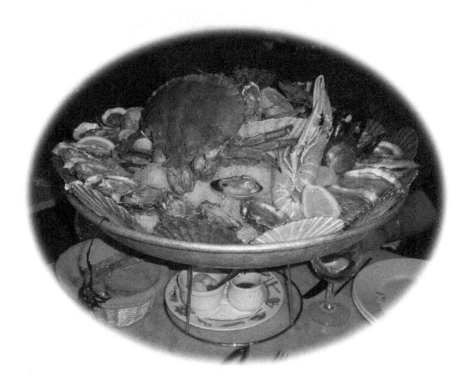

Aphrodisiacs and Science

'Scientia est potentia.'('Knowledge is Power.') – Latin

Aphrodisiacs can be roughly divided into **three main groups**, which either separately or in combination can assist in the enhancement and/or maintenance of healthy libido:

Physical – promoting blood circulation to the sexual organs, or trigger the body's own production of hormones.

Psychological – relaxing over stressed nervous system and muscles, and promoting good mood and sexual receptiveness.

Emotional – creating impulses to the brain via our senses like smell (perfumes, aromas, pheromones, body's secretions, sweat, etc), touch (gentle or painful, etc), taste (sweet, sour, bitter or mixed). vision (colours, level of light, pornographic images, etc), and hearing (hormone laden voices, music, rhythm, pitch, etc).

By experimenting with as many aphrodisiacs as possible, in various different combinations, you will be able to identify your own personal 'ultimate aphrodisiac' and reward yourself with lots of pleasurable moments. In essence, the selection of aprohrodisiacs is very simple – what doesn't appeal to your senses is not good for you!

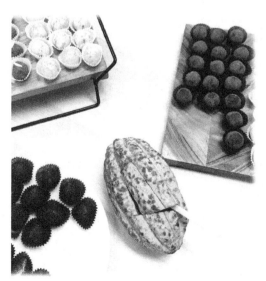

Please note:

Aphrodisiacs will not be able to help people with permanent physical or mental disabilities, chronic sickness or accidental loss of say, the testicles, etc. Like any other consumables, aphrodisiacs should be taken in moderation and, as has already been stated, it is advisable to consult your physician prior to experimenting with aphrodisiacs.

You can be assured that it's not just you and me who are interested in discovering the magic of aphrodisiacs! Since early civilisations, people on all continents have put high value on their sexuality and hunted for the secret fountain of youth, which could preserve it.

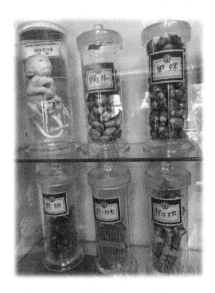

They have searched for the magic aids throughout the ages – barely leaving an animal or plant that has not been trialled as an aphrodisiac – and many have now been proven by science. From ancient medicinal texts to modern science, it's been shown that the sexual, physical and mental functions of all living creatures can be altered by certain bioactive compounds that are either synthesised by the body or absorbed from the outside. The misbalance of these compounds can also directly affect the physical, emotional or mental health vital for healthy libido. These compounds became known as aphrodisiacs, the natural remedies named after Aphrodite – the ancient Greek Goddess of love, beauty, pleasure, and procreation.

History is full of examples where aphrodisiacs were used to start wars or seduce lovers, gain riches, keep harem women content, or to enhance, prolong, reclaim sexual pleasures or even to vindicate ex-spouse. Like Josephine, who after learning about Napoleon's decision to divorce her, deliberately

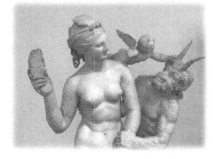

stained carved wood in her bedroom with her favourite potent musk oil perfume (originally obtained from the abdominal glands of the male musk deer), which for many years triggered Napoleon's memories of the hot love they had together and affected his sexual performance with his new wife. Or Cleopatra, who skillfully played with exquisite fragrances and herbs to create magic aphrodisiac effects on her lovers. Like mix of orange-blossom oil, animal-like musky patchouli and ambergris, known to reduce anxiety connected with sex, raise sensuality, enhance sexual longing and cravings for sensual euphoria.

It is known, that well-to-do ancient Greeks customary attended parties, which were held at the specially designed androns (rooms for men), where they were entertained by male and female objects of their desire - hetairai (slave mistresses). There they enjoyed music and poetry, participated in group sex, held philosophical debates and consumed aphrodisiacs with their food and wine. During those times creative herbalists, alchemists, artists, musicians, poets and cooks, who could manipulate human senses by using natural remedies, were in high demand. At the specially designed Aphrodite temples the most beautiful prostitutes armed with knowledge of sexual stimulants plied their ancient trade among the exquisite coloured marble statues.

Long before science discovered pheromones in the 1980s, people instinctively used the mysterious power of their unique smellprint by slipping their soiled underwear into the pockets or under the pillows of their lovers.

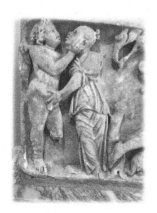

In order to enhance their lover's affection, the Middle Ages paramours gave to each other with lockets filled with their hair as an enticing fragrant amulet.

People searched all over earth and sea for hidden remedies which could help them to preserve or regain the pleasure of passion, or push their sexual limitations to new heights by making their blood boil with desire!

No stone was left unturned ... plants, seeds, animals, insects, minerals, chemical substances, poisons, spices, excrement, blood, bones, hearts, smelly animal glands, internal organs, genitals, horns, the embryos of living creatures, precious metals and stones, human sperm and menstrual blood

They also often resorted to consuming anything that simply resembled sexual organs or secreted milky juices, or animals that seemed to display hypoactive sexual desire, such as sparrows, bulls, roosters, rabbits, deer, horses and crocodiles, tigers, rhinoceros and poisonous snakes, just to name a few. All have been trialed as aphrodisiac in foods, amulets, witchcraft and love potions.

Both rich and poor – whether alchemist or uneducated peasant – often risked their lives by experimenting with countless bizarre and even dangerous substances thought to be aphrodisiacs. Substantial prices were paid for anything that worked as an aphrodisiac, conversely, if it did not work, the so-called 'aphrodisiacs' were never used again. Many died in the process, but those who found real ones made a fortune!

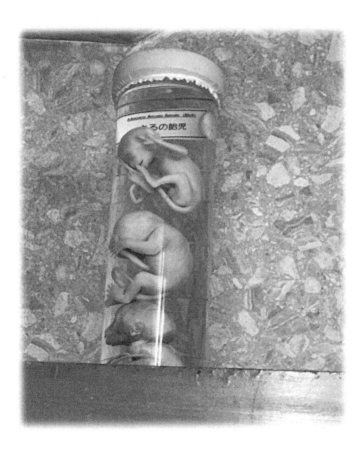

Many ancient aphrodisiacs have now been explained and substantiated by the science. For example, we know why protein foods (meat, poultry, seafood, eggs, beans or nuts) are high in amino acids , which influence levels of neurotransmitters like dopamine, seratonin, norepinephrine and endorphins responsible for sensual emotions such as ecstasy, euphoria, elation and sexual desire.

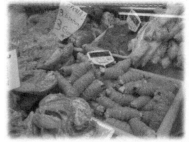

The mysterious effectiviness of many unusual aphrodisiacs discovered by our ancestors had now been explained. Like birds nests, which made by sea swallows from their saliva mixed with edible seaweed leaves, rich in the phosphrous spawn of fish.

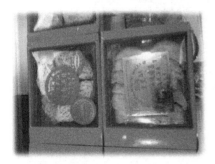

While in China, my husband and I experienced the powerful action of delightful increased desire after eating fabulously expensive birds-nest soup, however we soon learned that too much of this special dish can produce a toxic reaction.

Same applies to alcohol, which in small quantities can produce a pleasant stimulating effect and add zest to sex or fire amorous appetites, while its over-indulgence is known to produce anti-aphrodisiac effects, including disappointment of temporary impotence despite a possible strong desire.

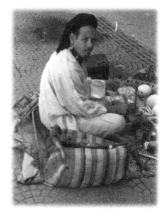

There are many aphrodisiacs on offer, that claim to be effective, however one should be very careful of consuming unknown to them substances. Few years ago we spoted in Morocco a street vendor, who sold some homemade sex stimulating electuaries made of honey, saffron, cinnamon, nutmeg, cloves, cubeb pepper and very dangerous for internal consumption secretions of cantharides - blister beetles.

There are also many other than food effective aphrodisiacs, which work through our senses of smell, touch, sight, etc. Like erotic images, fragrances, sensual manipulation, dancing and music, which have also been used for thousands of years to reinforce sexual desire and arouse responsiviness to a lover's advances and which will be featured in my next book.

The powerful effects of many aphrodisiacs experienced by my husband and I, cannot be denied. I hope that this book will inspire you to take action and bring that most enjoyable carnal happiness back into your live!

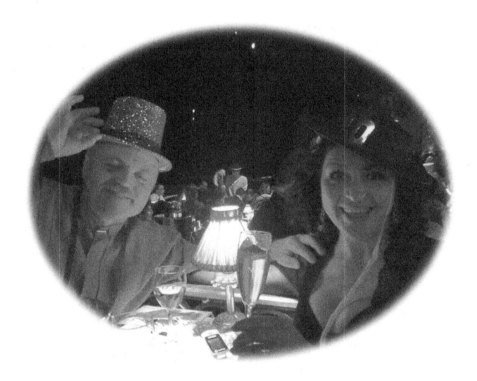

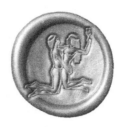

About the Recipes

'He, who experiments the most – wins!' - Old saying

Throughout thirty plus years of hunting for aphrodisiacs, I discovered many effective powerful remedies and numerous legendary and traditional folk recipes, often based on myths and lore, which fortunately for us, were handed down verbally from one generation to another. However not every recipe will be suitable for everyone.

There is an old saying – 'He, who experiments the most – wins! Please use provided in this book recipes and preparation technics, but feel absolutely free to modify them to suit your tastes. And one more thing – smile more often, as stress is the biggest ENEMY of aphrodisiacs.

Most of the recipes my husband and I tried out personally, to satisfy our curiosity and to be able to validate their effectiveness. Part of the appeal of these recipes is that they hold memories of the past, enabling us to have a little taste of the ancient cookery and magic from those times, as well as to experience the power of culinary orgasms from traditional or created by the great chefs dishes that have been used in witchcraft, sacred rituals and festivals.

While it is fun to experiment, prepare and experience these recipes, special attention must be paid to dosages, preparation methods and the quality of ingredients. But most importantly, that aphrodisiacs are not a magic bullet – they are only ingredients, which you will need to work with in order to live your dream-life. I'm tossing you the keys, so you can test drive aphrodisiacs! All you need is just two things to ramp your life FAST - explore and identify those ingredients, which work for you. So you can execute your dream FAST without having to jerk around and get frustrated with strange substances, diets, drugs, chemical stimulants, or fuss.

Every chapter of this book ends with a legend, which can make great table topics and provoke very interesting conversations at your dinner parties. These entertaining legends and folktales are bejewelled with some unexpected humorous twists of historical facts, such as when aphrodisiac recipes were used by famous figures to gain power, seduce lovers, pursue fame or simply prolong sexual pleasures. For example, the Russian tsar – Peter the Great – was tricked into marriage by the peasant girl Martha, who used an aphrodisiac to ignite the tsar's passion, while King Solomon seduced the Queen of Sheba with erotic poems and a love potion.

Then there are the stories of famous women, such as Queen Cleopatra, Josephine Bonaparte, or Madame de Pompadour, who used aphrodisiacs to conquer men's hearts and enjoy the benefits of their power. These titillating topics will fill your dinner parties with plenty of fun, tasty experience and delicious wickedness!

Open your mind and get your sexual energy running NOW.

Are you up to the challenge?

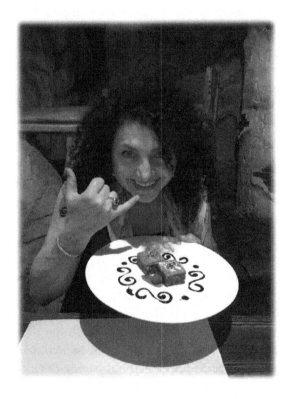

For more information and recipes,
go to https://www.aphrodisiacsexpert.com/aphrodisiacs-expert-blog/

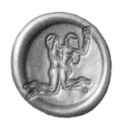

Aphrodisiac Sources

Due to high demand and great value of aphrodisiacs, some traders might offer totally useless, and even hazardous substances, or substances that produce dangerous or an anti-aphrodisiac effects. So always ensure the authenticity and proper strength of your aphrodisiacs by sourcing them from reputable places.

It's important to be aware that if you choose to substitute ingredients or their quantities, your aphrodisiac recipe might not produce desired effects, as there is a very fine line between pleasure and pain, energy and relaxtion, sexual desire and the desire to sleep.

Many aphrodisiacs can be simply foraged, however unless you have solid knowledge of plant and minerals lore, it is advisable that you get your aphrodisiacs from reputible sources, rather than gathering them by yourself in the wild. Some aphrodisiac plants can be easily grown in your own garden, however their strength will depend on the environmental conditions, soil, time of harvests and other components. Unless you have this special knowledge, you might jeopardize your health or be disappointed.

Betel Nut – Myanmar

Areca catechu (Latin) or Areca Nut

(The areca nut is also known as the betel nut since it is often chewed along with the leaf of the betel plant.)

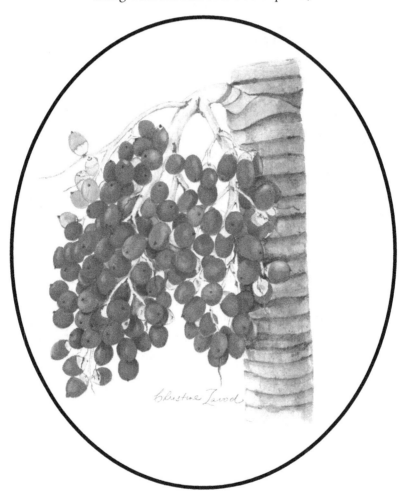

Chewing areca nut is known to elevate mood and sexuality as in combination with lime (calcium oxide) and betel leaf (contains chemical compounds like, chavicol, cadinene and chavibetol), it produces arecoline oil - a mild central nervous system stimulant, which gets released from the nut into saliva.   *Dr. V.L.Zeltser*

My gardener Arjun, whose 'green thumb' and great persistence turned my drought-suffering garden into a luscious Garden of Eden, migrated to Australia from Myanmar (formerly Burma) with his family and kids. His teeth had a dark red tint, but I never dared to ask him why, until one day it came up in conversation with him about my favourite subject -aphrodisiacs.

Pointing at his stained teeth, the very shy Arjun happily explained that it came from chewing traditional Burmese 'paan', which was sometimes called 'betel quid' or 'paan paan'. It is made of areca palm nut, slaked lime and betel leaves, with the addition of some other ingredients. He assured me that it was safe, and that he used it on a regular basis to help him relax and feel happy, and to make his wife happy in bed.

Noticing that I was interested in the subject, Arjun produced from his pocket a small triangular bundle wrapped in silver foil and offered it for me to try. I probably looked hesitant, as Arjun demonstratively pulled the foil off the parcel which was wrapped in a greenish leaf, and put it behind his cheek. After a minute or so, he chewed and spat out red coloured saliva on the grass, saying that it was good for the plants as well. He also told me that his family and everyone in Burma chews paan daily.

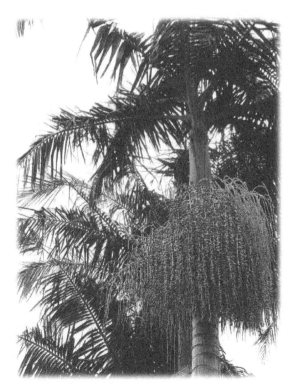

I began to research the subject, and found that the tradition came from India, where this symbol of royalty was used for hundreds of years as an effective mood and sex stimulant. Every family in Burma has their own favourite paan recipe, which is usually passed from parent to child.

The next week Arjun brought me a small paan, made from a recipe his wife Umi inherited from her great-grandmother, who was the most famous paan-maker in their village, and who made paans for newlyweds to promote excitement and sexual responsiveness. This special paan was wrapped in real gold foil made by the skilled gold-beaters of Myanmar. In Burma these shiny foils (gold leaves) are usually saved by the groom, who is expected to bring them to the temple the morning after the wedding night, and attach them to the statue of Buddha and pray for prosperity and fertility.

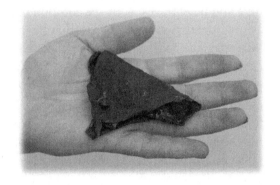

It wasn't polite for me to refuse Arjun's treat and reluctantly I put it into my mouth. He happily instructed me to place it behind my cheek and start slowly chewing after it would get wet with saliva. The paan had a strange subtle yet complex, grassy, bitter-sweet and peppery taste, with notes of liquorice and roses at the same time. Some ingredients, affected by my saliva, created a soft and pleasant burning sensation in my mouth. My face and ears reddened, and I felt a pleasant soft pulsation in my genitals. In a few minutes, my whole body and mind felt elated, content and sexually alert. I was advised to spit out the red saliva.

While I diligently chewed and spat this newly discovered aphrodisiac treat, I remembered that as a child I saw green saliva stains on the footpaths in Uzbekistan, where they used a pungent green snuff called 'nasvay'. This mix of powdered tobacco, wood ash and calcium hydrate, with a very powerful smell of hay, was traditionally used by the Uzbeks, who kept it for hours under their lower lip. While this snuff was very popular in Middle Asia and Turkey as a stimulant and aphrodisiac, it was banned in Tsarist Russia, where users of 'barbarian' snuff faced jail time in Siberia. A few years later, while in Sweden, I also spotted another stimulant, known since the early eighteen century as 'snus'. It was made of made of tobacco, salt and sodium carbonate and came in small teabags, which Swedes kept for extended periods in their upper lip.

This delightful encounter prompted our expedition to Myanmar – one of the least visited Southeast Asian countries – where I was hoping to unearth local secrets and experience the powers of the betel nut.

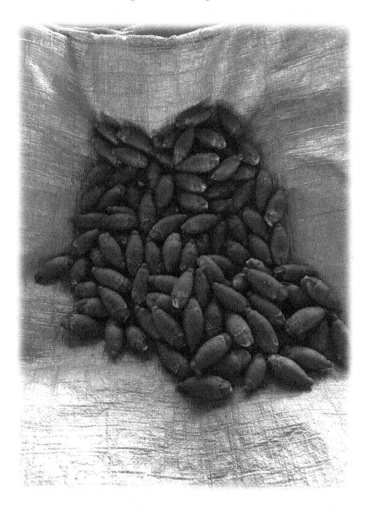

Further research revealed that approximately 450 million people chew betel nut, which is the seed of a medium-sized lush tropical palm (Areca catechu) often planted around palaces and parks in India and Southeast Asia. The nuts are consumed fresh, dried, boiled, baked, roasted or cured. The psychoactive substance in these nuts works similarly to nicotine, alcohol or caffeine, producing a surge of happiness and a mildly euphoric, stimulating effect with feelings of wellbeing and sociability. Its magic usually starts with a light biting-like sensation in the throat, followed by pleasant feelings of physical excitement and slight drowsiness.

The word 'paan' derives from the Sanskrit word 'parna' meaning 'leaf'. It is a popular cultural tradition in Southeast Asian countries to chew chopped-up areca seeds wrapped in betel leaves. Paan has many variations, as people tend to create their own recipes by adding ingredients according to their own taste, like rose-petal jam, cardamom, candied fruit, date paste, shredded coconut, peanut butter, honey, chocolate, tobacco, etc.

Lime paste, calcium hydroxide mixed with some water, locally known as choona, is commonly added to bind ingredients to betel leaves, which are traditionally folded into tight small triangles. This paste empowers the release of alkaloids and high-inducing chemicals from the betel leaves and sliced areca nuts into human saliva, which can be either spat out or swallowed.

Nobody knows for sure who invented paan, however it is well-documented that this addictive and euphoria-inducing treat had been used for centuries for its effective hallucinogenic and psychoactive properties at weddings and religious ceremonies, and as a legally permitted recreational drug.

When we arrived in mysterious Yangon, the capital of Myanmar, we noticed the smiles of almost all local people were permanently stained by red pigment. Totally devoted to their traditions and Buddhism, they live in houses made of bamboo, eat fermented tea leaves called 'lahpet', indulge by chewing paans, talk to the spirits of their ancestors daily, and keep them happy with gifts.

Most of the men prefer wearing traditional skirts to pants and carry umbrellas to protect themselves from the sun. Some of them have secret protective tattoos on their backs, made by praying monks armed with traditional long needles and ink. Women paint their faces with paste made of tanaka (jungle tree bark).

The footpaths and most of the streets are stained with red spit produced by thousands of people with puffy cheeks and hazy eyes, chewing paans. The saliva is spat out almost everywhere, with the exception of on public transport, where it's ceremoniously done into small plastic bags provided by the driver.

Everyone in this busy megalopolis seemed to be extra courteous, polite and curious seeing a Caucasian woman interested in paans. Tired of telling hundreds of total strangers 'where we were from', my husband made a little sign that said 'Australia', which we kept above our heads – however, it did not help as not many could read English.

Bustling rundown colonial streets downtown were filled with hundreds of competing paan vendors, who displayed their colourful ingredients, unusual bottles with aromatic essences, chopped-up stripy betel nuts, green heart-shaped leaves, herbs, candied fruit and paans made to their own unique recipes. The prices varied here from one to ten cents per piece.

Most paan vendors happily gave me their best paans free of charge, as I seemed to attract the attention of the crowds at their stalls. After having two sweet paans, I experienced a high feeling of being slightly dizzy, but very happy, relaxed, sensual and content. This feeling lasted for approximately two hours.

Using 'Google Translate', a friendly paan vendor told me that he was an ex-poppy farmer, who suffered a loss of sustainable income when opium bans were implemented in Burma under international pressure. While Myanmar produces the world's best precious stones such as rubies, sapphires, pearls and jade, it is also the world's second largest producer of opium. I suddenly realised that the paans, which were still in my mouth, could contain traces of opium.

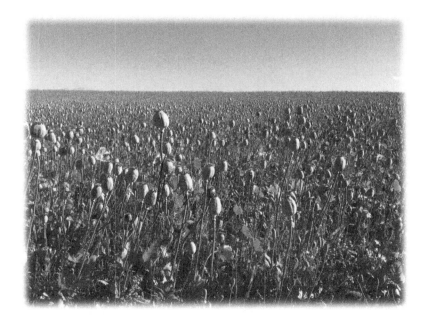

A few years later while researching ashwagandha in Nepal, I came across paan made with opium, which confirmed my suspicions. Then, while in Cambodia, we tried paans made with scallops, which were sold as powerful trance-generating aphrodisiacs.

I visited my gardener's sister Hayma, who lived with her family of six in a house constructed from rusted-out corrugated iron sheets in one of Yangon's poorest suburbs. They came here from the Golden Triangle after their poppy farm was sold to a large company. Hayma's husband was away on monk's duty, which every Burmese man has to do at least once in his lifetime. My husband thought it was a great excuse for any man to escape the house legally and have his wife feel good about it!

After receiving the gifts we had brought for her and her family from Australia, Hayma agreed to prepare some aphrodisiac paans for us without any opium, which her husband sold in the streets.

To end our Burmese aphrodisiac adventure, my husband and I had two paans each, one after another, which tinted our teeth and produced two hours of pleasant sexual excitement and delicious cheerfulness.

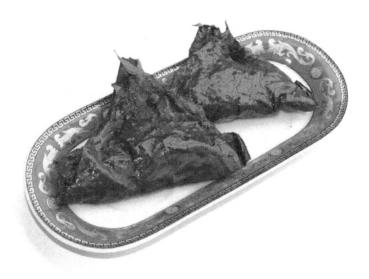

Hayma's Paan

6 fresh betel leaves (these leaves have a perfect heart shape and
are considered to be the feminine part of the paan)

2g dried mint leaves, rubbed

2 teaspoons of rose-petal or mango jam

10-12 shavings (approx 30g) of areca nut, shaved or crushed

6g choona (lime powder)

4 pods cardamom, crushed

6g fenugreek seed, powdered

6g ashwangandha root, powdered

Serves 6

Mix lime powder with cold water into a soft paste, and spread on the
flattened large betel leaves. Mix rose-petal or mango jam with mint and
roasted fenugreek powders (one of my favourite aphrodisiacs which,
since antiquity, has been used in love recipes, as it contains gentle sex
stimulating chemicals and an unusual delightful flavour, sweet and
nutty, with slightly bitter undertones). Spread this mixture on the leaves
and place shavings of betel nut and a pinch of crushed cardamom pods
on their edges, then carefully fold each leaf, forming six tight triangle
parcels. Make sure that all ingredients are locked inside. Wrap each quid
(paan) in foil. Keep refrigerated.

Enjoy this mild sensual stimulant by chewing it and spitting out red
saliva in a bowl. Laugh at the red-stained smile and be delighted by this
sensual experience.

But please also note, offering paan to a person from Melanesia might
be considered to be a sign of your sexual desire for that person!

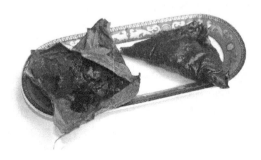

Legend: Antique Viagra Tea

Suleiman the Magnificent - the greatest and richest ruler of the Ottoman Empire, was known as a true connoisseur of food, art, jewellery and beautiful women. His royal harem contained over 300 of the most gorgeous women from all over the world.

Naturally, to enjoy these riches, he required extra stamina. However, the Sultan's love bedchamber was not being used, and everyone was worried for their future as there was no heir to the throne. Mahidevran, one of the Sultan's concubines, given to him by a Persian merchant as a gift, happened to be the niece of the famous alchemist Mansur ibn Ilyas and was privy to medicinal herbs. She ordered merchants to bring secret herbs from India and the Far East, from which she made a potent love-tea. After convincing the Sultan's vizier about its efficacy, she served it to the sultan … and the rest is history!

Her love-brew helped Suleiman to live his dreams and soon Mahidevran gave birth to a healthy son Şehzade Mustafa – the future heir of Suleiman's throne. Suleiman married Mahidevran, who became known as Gülbahar – the 'Rose of Spring'. The Sultan continued drinking the tea and maintained his sexual appetite even in his old age, which resulted in him fathering more than 300 children and for that reaknown in history as Suleiman the Magnificent.

Recipe:

2 tablespoons of galangal root, freshly grated

1 Tibetan pi-pi-ling pepper (long pepper)

10ml rosewater or orange-blossom water

1 areca nut, sliced

4 teaspoons of fresh cream

5 tablespoons of honey, cold pressed

3g powdered sea pearl (or mother pearl)

4 cups of spring or filtered water (or red wine)

Combine all ingredients in the pot and whisk them together until the honey dissolves. Cover and let simmer for ten minutes. Pour liquid into a teapot and serve in small tea cups by pouring liquid through the sieve. This tea delights the senses with its unusual flavours, relaxes and provokes luscious feelings of happiness, lust and enhanced sexual responsiveness.

Zallouh - Israel

Ferula hermonis (Latin), Arabian Viagra

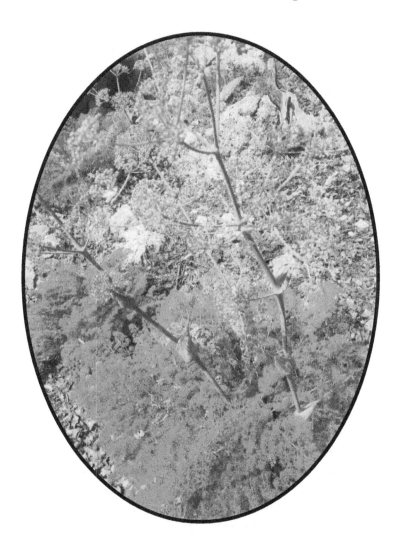

This bitter root had been used since antiquity to enhance libido for men and women. Its unique composition of minerals, vitamins and crude oil turns this plant into perfect agent for boosting sexual function and adding extra pleasure to amorous activity.   *Dr. V.L.Zeltser*

After holidaying in Israel, our family friends, who were aware of my life obsession with aphrodisiacs, told me that they had come across very expensive honey sold in Tel Aviv as a sexual stimulant. It was produced from the flowers of the rare native aphrodisiac plant called 'zallouh'. Later I found it for sale online in 340g jars at US$149.99 each, which triggered further research.

It took me to King Solomon, who – in his erotic love verses, 'The Song of Songs' – attributed his sexual powers to an aphrodisiac plant called 'dudaïm', which grew on the holy slopes of Mount Hermon. Further investigation proved that, since ancient times, villagers of Lebanon and Syria collected the potent herb from Mount Hermon, which they called 'shirsh zallouh', and which was used as a libido stimulant for both sexes. It had an extraordinarily positive effect on men with erectile problems and was even given to sheep to stimulate reproduction.

Pharmacists in modern Lebanon and Syria sell concoctions from hairy zallouh root, marketing them as natural Arabian viagra with no side effects. Dried, pounded, pulverised, extracted in water or oil, the root is usually administered mixed with tea, juice or milk. The Latin name of zallouh, *ferula hermonis*, refers to its species and origin – Mount Hermon!

Thus it was not unreasonable of me to suspect that King Solomon's mysterious aphrodisiac dudaïm, was in fact, zallouh. Therefore, it was time we went on a zallouh quest to Israel!

Ori, a local botanist and historian, had led our expedition to the high alpine meadow of the massive Mount Hermon (*Har Hermon* in Hebrew), which also serves as a border between Syria, Israel and Lebanon. The holy mountain is the only place on earth where ferula harmonis, locally known as zallouh, still grows in the wild.

Signs along the fence on the slopes of the mountain warned us about possible minefields, however Ori assured us that it was safe to walk around the area, as he frequently walked there with his dog.

For thousands of years locals used zallouh as an aphrodisiac, so one can only marvel that despite its popularity it has survived in the wild till now. The Arabs on the other side of the mountain cultivate and commercially process it, selling the plant as 'natural viagra', which has resulted in wild zallouh being almost extinct on their side of the mountain.

According to Ori, the same wild zallouh plants can be harvested indefinitely, as long as the plant is not uprooted. Experienced zallouh foragers do not take out the whole plant, but dig out only a few outer roots leaving the inner roots intact. This technique allows the plant to re-establish itself in a few years and produce new roots.

In my opinion, zallouh should be grown in large quantities all over Mount Hermon and given to all people in the Middle East for free, as I believe that sexually satisfied people are more open to happiness, love and peace.

And there it was – the legendary zallouh! A small modest shrub with thin mustard-like foliage and tiny pale umbrellas of pink or yellow flowers covered with local bees attracted by the strong honey aroma.

We were not allowed to harvest any plants on the holy mountain due to government regulations, which only permit the harvesting of zallouh at certain times of the year.

As a historian, Ori claimed to have cracked King Solomon's famous love-wine recipe, and he was happy to share it with us for a fee. I thought that it would be fun to try, and agreed.

The following love-wine recipe is allegedly attributed to King Solomon. Ori prepared it from dried zallouh roots, which we purchased at the Tel Aviv central market. Excited, Ori got on with the preparations while telling us about some of the interesting historical events from the life of King Solomon.

In 967 BCE King Solomon, the son of the famous King David, inherited his vast kingdom that stretched from the Euphrates River in the north to Egypt. Surrounded by many fearsome neighbours ready to kill and rob his kingdom, Solomon, who was well-educated and knowledgeable in alchemy and pharmacopeia, decided to secure his empire's political stability through love instead of battle.

Thus, the wise man ended up marrying 700 daughters of his neighbours, as well as collecting 305 exotic and beautiful concubines. But the real phenomenon is that all his women really loved him. How did he do that?!

The legend says that the wisest and the richest king of antiquity created an amazing aphrodisiac love-wine, which allegedly produced astonishing amorous effects on his women and strengthened his own sexual energy beyond belief. Having a romantic nature, he gave them wine and spoiled each of his women with lavish gifts and erotic love verses, known to us as 'The Song of Songs'.

Solomon's fame travelled faster than the wind, until it reached the ears of the beautiful and most-celebrated southern Arabian queen – Sheba. Curious, she sent to the king many presents in exchange for the recipe of his love-wine, but the wisest of men did not agree to give away his secret. Instead, he invited her to come over and share the magic wine with him.

> '... *Show me your true charms, my black crown diamond!*
> *Spin my head with the excitingly delightful aroma of your loins,*
> *Like an aphrodisiac from Mount Hermon!'*

The most beautiful 'Black Diamond' of King Solomon's crown, the Queen of Sheba, fell in love with the king – even more than she did with his magic wine. To honour this amazing event, in 1,000 BCE King Solomon commissioned a temple to be built at the foot of Mount Hermon.

The flower of this union was their son Menelik, who later inherited his mother's throne and became the great ruler of Sheba. Solomon's blood line has continued to this day, with all rulers of Ethiopia believed to be directly descended from King Solomon and the Queen of Sheba.

My husband and I enjoyed Ori's aphrodisiac love-wine, despite the fact that it didn't produce any erotic dreams or magic by turning my husband into the King of Judea or me into his hot Black Diamond. Perhaps Ori's formula needs to be fine-tuned.

Ori's Love-Wine

1 bottle of sweet red kosher wine made from the grapes of
Mount Carmel

100g zallouh root, fresh (or 40g, dried and pounded in the
mortar then reconstituted in 5 tablespoons of warm filtered water
overnight before cooking)

100g coriander seeds, finely cracked just before cooking

10 fresh basil leaves (or ½ teaspoon of dried leaves)

¼ lemon, zested

300ml filtered water

Place all ingredients, except the wine, in a clean pot, stir, cover with lid
and let simmer for two hours. Let the pot stand in a cool dark place for
twenty-four hours. Strain liquid through a fine sieve and mix with wine.
Pour into a dark glass bottle with tight cap. Store in a cool dark place.
Enjoy the bitter-sweet taste of love and magic.

Back home, I used double the amount of recommended powdered
zallouh in my recipe, which created a pleasing libido-stimulating effect
for my husband and I.

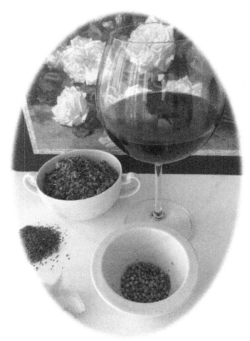

Wormwood - Switzerland

Artemisia absinthium (Latin) – Grand Wormwood

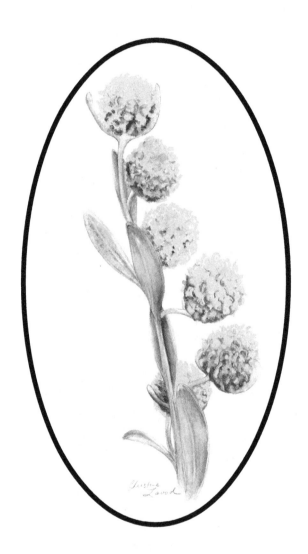

This plant contains codeine-like analgesic narcotic compound, which can be dangerous in large quantities. It is known to induce a dreamy state conductive to creativity by suppressing feelings of anxiety and pain.

Dr. V.L.Zeltser

This aphrodisiac adventure was triggered by a bottle of green liqueur known as 'absinthe', given to me as a birthday gift by my young friend, Natalie. There was a little booklet attached to the bottle, alerting me to its wicked reputation and ceremonial drinking customs. The main ingredient of the liqueur was a plant with the unappetising name of 'wormwood', which had been known to produce 'magic' – hallucinogenic – experiences, and was featured as an ingredient in love potions and rituals in many European and Asian cultures.

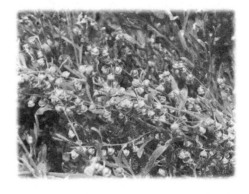

Further research revealed that this liqueur was popular among the French bohemians of the eighteenth to twentieth centuries. Philosophers, painters and musicians such as Ernest Hemingway, Henri de Toulouse-Lautrec, Amedeo Modigliani, Pablo Picasso, Vincent van Gogh, Oscar Wilde, Edgar Allan Poe and Lord Byron, just to name a few, were among its devotees.

This highly alcoholic liqueur, infused with hallucinogenic plant, miraculously inspired generations of talented people by provoking strong surges of sexual energy and creativity. However, its regular use was known to aggravate adverse mental health effects, cause violent crimes and social disorder. Thus it was abandoned in France and other countries, only to be revived two hundred years later without its main active ingredient – wormwood.

Despite this fact, my husband and I were keen to experience its magic – however, we were greatly disappointed when, after imbibing the bitter-sweet liqueur with its licorice undertones, we only felt the intoxicating effect of the alcohol, and nothing more.

Further research revealed that the wormwood plant contains thujone – a fragrant substance found in several edible plants including commonly used herbs such as tarragon and sage. This chemical, which gives absinthe its hallucinogenic reputation, can be toxic, especially if used regularly in high doses.

In medieval times, this plant was used in magic ceremonies and witchcraft, as well as medically, to prompt abortions, deal with intestinal worms and to settle stomach illnesses. Producing an intoxicating smoke, wormwood – a potent relative of the daisy – was also used in rituals to expel demons and to cause a state of sexual excitement and mild euphoria. There are also many folk tales and legends where wormwood was used to help people achieve success with their desired love target.

Naturally, we wanted to investigate wormwood further – particularly from where it originated historically – the luscious wilderness of the alpine Jura Mountains, Western Switzerland.

La Chaux-de-Fonds is an old Swiss city at an altitude of 1,000 metres in the region of Neuchâtel in the Jura Mountains, a few kilometres south of the French border and our cozy room at the Farmhouse B&B.

We were lucky to engage a charismatic local botanist, Jorgen, as our guide. He spoke favourably about wormwood and its role in the lives of indigenous Swiss people, who since antiquity have used wormwood as a medicinal plant, a spice for beer and wine, an amulet against witchcraft and, most importantly, as a mysterious love-inducing remedy – which he arranged to be prepared for us by the local seventy-five-year-old witch Emma.

According to Jorgen, there are many species of wormwood that grow in the Swiss Alps, however the only really potent one is Artemisia absinthium. As was the case in many of the destinations we had visited on our aphrodisiac journey, overharvesting had caused the plants – including wormwood – to hide on the higher rocky areas of the almost vertical cliffs, protected by gravity against greedy foragers. Using alpinists' gear we climbed up the steep cliff and there it was – the magnificent wormwood, happily-growing in abundance – protected, according to the ancient Greek myth, by Artemis, goddess of the hunt and wilderness.

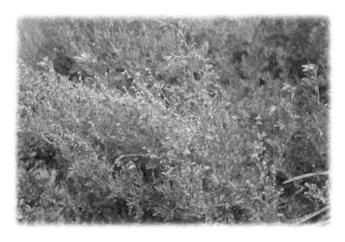

The intricate, pale-green leaves with clusters of small greenish-yellow flowers projected something mystical. Mesmerised, and catching my breath, I stood there for some time just admiring the bushes, which beautifully decorated the rocky landscape, while Jorgen demonstrated how to snap off the wormwood flowers and leaves without causing damage to the plant. After collecting a small bag of leaves and flowers, we descended to the picturesque alpine village set in a green valley, and went to see Emma, the witch, who happened to be Jorgen's grandmother!

She lived in a distinctively traditional Swiss chalet with wooden stairs on the outside of the house, which reached the first floor's geranium-decorated balcony.

Dressed in a dirndl – a traditional dress – the grey-haired Emma welcomed us with her famous love-potion drink. She seemed to be overwhelmed by our interest in her skills. While resting on her soft, velvet armchairs and sipping her delicious schnapps made of dried cherries, wormwood and other spices, we listened to Jorgen, as he translated her story.

Emma's grandmother Agatha had a long, ugly nose and could not find any man to marry. Tired by her neighbours' gossip and parents' naggings, the thirty-five-year-old woman went to see the local witch, who made her a wormwood love potion. Evidently it worked, as the first man who tried the potion from Agatha's hands married her. More so, every summer thereafter she gave birth to a child.

Local villagers, encouraged by Agatha's success, came up with an interesting custom, which often resulted in marriage proposals. Going from one farmhouse to another, the bachelors visited unmarried farmers' daughters. At each farm, they drank one glass of love potion prepared by the maiden, under the watchful eye of the local witch, and inevitably fell in love with one girl – or another.

This recipe had been in Emma's family for over a hundred years, and unfortunately she could not give it to us. Teasingly, Jorgen reminded her about her 'capuns' – Swiss dumplings prepared with dough and pieces of dried meat, rolled in a chard leaf and covered with grated cheese, and served in broth – which had also made her famous among the locals, for their aphrodisiac effects. The kindly witch agreed to cook her capuns for us and share the recipe, which was based on the traditional local recipe, but with a twist.

Her love potion slowly worked its magic on our moods and our bodies, tired by the mountain climbing. Tempting aromas coming from Emma's kitchen teased our senses and heightened our excitement for what was to come. This feeling was intensified when Jorgen explained that there was ritual for eating capuns, and that diners who could not fit the whole capun in their mouth had to kiss their neighbour!

Eventually the magnificent capuns were served, accompanied by yet more schnapps. Our dinner was filled with laughter, especially when my husband decided to change his seat after kissing old Emma a number of times.

The real power of Emma's delicious and cheesy capuns became obvious within an hour of finishing the dinner, when the dark Swiss mountain sky suddenly sparkled with millions of brilliant stars.

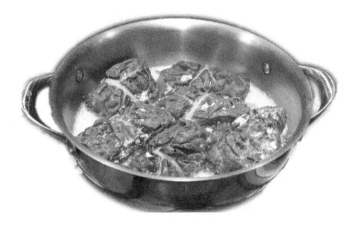

Emma's Capuns

400g wholemeal flour

3 whole eggs

500ml water

1 litre milk, fresh

Salt to taste

Black pepper ground, to taste

400g cubed air-dried beef (dry-cured ham or salami can be used instead)

10g parsley, chopped

20g fresh wormwood leaves, chopped (or one teaspoon dried)

50g dried wormwood flowers

10g chives, chopped

12 fresh Swiss chard or silver beet leaves, stems removed, washed and patted dry

1 litre vegetable stock

50g butter

100g diced bacon

200g grated yellow cheese, preferably from the Swiss Alpine region

Serves 4

Place flour into a large bowl, add eggs, water, salt and pepper, and knead until the dough is firm and smooth, using some butter if it is too sticky. Cover and let it rest. Combine dough with cubed air-dried meat, chopped chives, parsley and wormwood leaves, and knead again until all ingredients are evenly distributed. Separate the dough mixture into twelve even portions, and form capuns by wrapping chard leaves tightly around the filling.

Combine milk and vegetable stock in a shallow pot and bring to simmer, then carefully add capuns and cook them gently on a low heat for about ten minutes. Fry diced bacon with butter. When they are ready, put capuns carefully onto warm soup plates, pour even amounts of liquid over them, and generously decorate with golden bacon pieces, grated cheese and wormwood flowers.

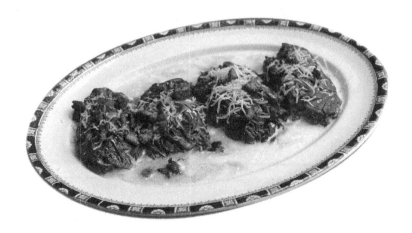

Jakub's Recipe

This wormwood recipe comes from the Czech Republic. It was prepared by herbalist Jakob, who was foraging for wormwood by the side of the road when we drove past a small village in the Alps near Prague.

   3 tablespoons of brown sugar

   1 handful of pine pollen

   1 egg white

   1 glass of crushed ice (Jacob used real snow instead)

   ½ glass of filtered water

   80g wormwood leaves, dried and rubbed

   500ml vodka (Jacob used homemade grape wine spirit)

Place wormwood leaves into the pot, add water, cover with lid, and gently simmer for ten minutes. Take off the heat and mix in pine pollen. Let stand for fifteen minutes. Mix egg and sugar with fork till sugar dissolves. Strain wormwood liquid into a large glass bottle, add alcohol, and the egg and sugar mixture. Shake well to create a little froth and serve with ice (or snow). Sip slowly.

This beverage produces strong, long-lasting libido-awakening effects and creative inspiration, but only when consumed in small 30ml servings at a time.

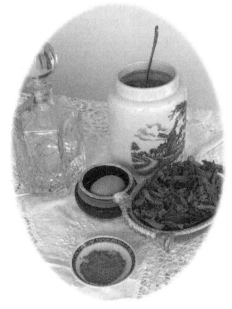

Legend: The King and His Love Chick

When the ambitious twenty-four-year-old Jeanne Antoinette Poisson was told by her husband that he could no longer support her obsession with jewellery, fashion, fine art and theatre, she decided to become a mistress of the richest person in France – King Louis XV.

According to the royal chronical, she managed to flirt King Louis XV into her bed in exchange for his lavish royal gifts and keep him interested for the next twenty years. How?

Realising that her modest beauty alone would not bring her ambitious plan to fruition, the smart lady resorted to aphrodisiacs, which an indulgent Louis was happy to experiment with, as long as they tasted nice. Thus, everything went to plan, and soon Jeanne Poisson became known as Madame de Pompadour, whose 'beloved' called her 'poulet d'amour' (Love Chick) and lavishly fulfilled her every wish until she died twenty years later.

Enjoy this finger-licking and lust-provoking dish, which will give you the opportunity to feel like a king!)

Recipe:

1 whole plump gutted chicken or pheasant, jointed
30g wormwood leaves and flowers, dried
4 cloves of garlic
1 tablespoon of olive oil
50g butter, unsalted
1 shallot, diced
100g baby spinach, cleaned
50g raw pine nut kernels
12 morel mushrooms
1 fresh truffle or 30ml of white truffle oil
100g of couscous (cracked wheat)
18 spears of green asparagus, fresh
1 grapefruit
½ bunch of dill
2 olives or red grapes
5 black peppercorns
3 teaspoons sea salt
Pinch of saffron
Pinch of barberries
100ml white wine

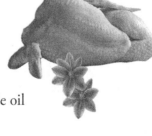

Serves 4

Chicken:

Pour glass of boiling water over the dried wormwood leaves. Cover with lid and let stand for fifteen minutes, then strain to separate leaves from the liquid. Keep both. Combine garlic and salt, and pound gradually adding soaked wormwood leaves, saffron and cracked black pepper. Add three teaspoons of cold pressed olive oil and mix well into a thick paste. Rub chicken inside and out with the paste. Cover and let rest at room temperature.

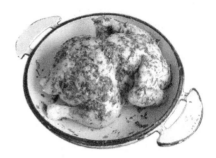

Stuffing:

Fry diced shallots and mushrooms in butter on low heat, until shallots turn golden. Take off the heat. Add to saved wormwood liquid salt, baby spinach, pine nuts and couscous. Mix well and cover with lid, and let stand till juices are absorbed. Mix in thinly sliced truffle or truffle oil. Carefully place stuffing mix into the chicken through the bottom. Wrap chicken in foil and pop on the baking dish. Roast in pre-heated (200°C) oven for thirty minutes. Take the foil off and let the skin roast till golden-brown (ten to fifteen minutes).

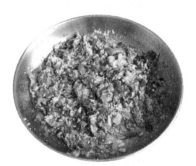

Garnish:

Clean asparagus of its woody skin and blanch in salted hot water for two minutes, then dip into icy-cold water to keep them crunchy. De-glaze baking dish with white wine. Reduce volume to half. Add grapefruit segments, let cook for one minute, then turn over and add barberries. Immediately take off the heat and use.

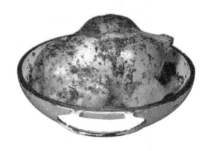

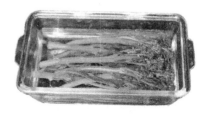

Presentation:

Arrange grapefruit segments on pre-heated plate between asparagus spears, creating an image of the sun. Place chicken in the centre of the sun and decorate it with dill, olives or grapes, according to your mood and imagination. Use reserved de-glazed juices as the dipping sauce for the chicken. Serve this exquisite dish to win the heart of your carnivore lover. If your lover happens to be vegetarian, replace chicken with pumpkin.

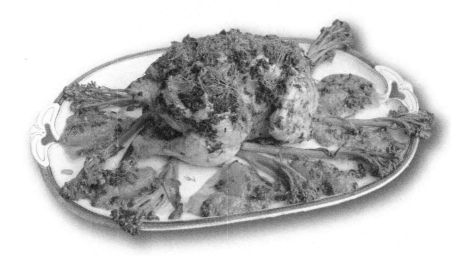

Kava – Hawaii

Piper methysticum (Latin), Kava or 'Awa

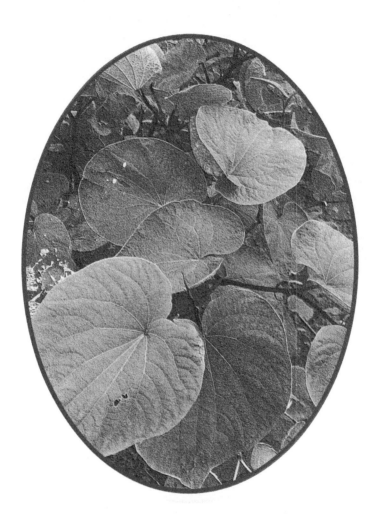

This plant contains active resinous chemical components called alpha pyrones, which in mild dozes can produce pleasant feelings of relaxation and euphoria while mental alertness is retained.

Dr. V.L.Zeltser

No one knows where kava originated from, however it seems that it travelled, through the centuries, all over the world. The ancient Egyptian papyrus, The Book of Aphrodisiacs, refers to the kava plant as an effective euphoria-inducing sexual stimulant used in sacred rituals devoted to Isis, the goddess of fertility and love.

In the last thirty years, I came across many places in Europe, the Americas and Oceania, where kava was consumed daily to stimulate sexuality by reducing stress. I tried many different kava recipes, mainly water-based root extractions, which admittedly had only a very mild effect on me, until I met Steven on the Hawaiian island of Kauai.

He moved there from Chicago, after falling in love with his future wife Alani, while they both studied naturopathy at the University of Illinois. Alani's family are native Hawaiians, who traditionally use kava as a medicine to alleviate anxiety, promote a heightened sense of well-being, increase of mental clarity, and as an aphrodisiac. Thus, the young naturopaths, armed with ancient kava recipes inherited by Alani from her family elders, decided to open the Kava Bar.

The bar was set in a luscious tropical garden full of flowers and bright-green kava plants, covered with their distinctive heart-shaped leaves. My husband ordered kava, which came served in cups made of coconut

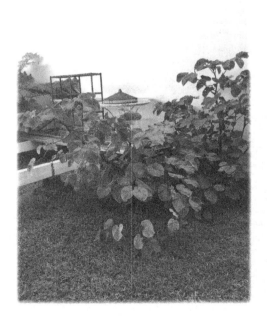

shell. I looked around and noticed that some of the kava plants were growing here in terracotta pots, while others were in the ground.

Steven explained that those in the pots were not cultivated, but were sourced from the ecologically clean Hawaiian wilderness, where in order to survive, plants synthesise more kavalactone compounds (desmethoxyyangonin), which are known to raise levels of dopamine and serotonin, slowly suppressing worry and anxiety, and making people more interested in social affairs and open to love.

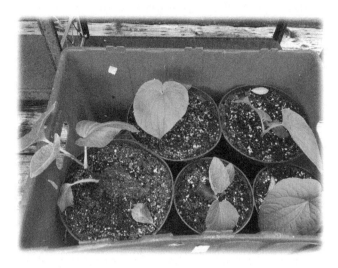

While enjoying Steven's kava, I told him about my many aphrodisiac experiences, and my disappointment with the effects of kava on previous occasions. A short while later, he introduced me to his wife Alani, and unexpectedly, invited my husband and I to experience the real aphrodisiac powers of kava by sharing a special luau (traditional feast) with them.

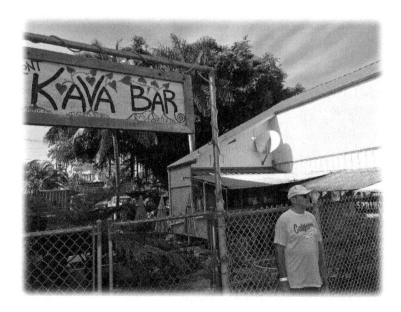

We walked behind the café and stopped under the shady tree in the typical Hawaiian outdoor kitchen with its imu (earth oven) in the centre. Alani picked six fresh kava leaves from the potted shrub nearby, and after washing and scrunching them, placed them into the huge teapot and topped it up with hot water.

After about ten minutes, the greenish tea was mixed with brown sugar, lemon and served in tall glasses with ice. It had a pleasant, balanced taste. Soon after drinking it, I became relaxed and cheerful, and felt totally at home in the strangers' house.

While Steven and my husband attended to building the fire in the imu according to the Hawaiian tradition, Alani and I got on with preparing the cooking vessel and ingredients.

I was in charge of cutting up meat, fish and onions into cubes, while Alani washed and cleaned taro and ti leaves. She skilfully removed ribs from the back of the leaves, turning them into soft wraps, which she competently fashioned into a sort of bowl or a large nest, which was meant to be used as the cooking vessel.

Peeled and finely chopped kava roots were mixed with cubed onions, cassava, meat, fish, and spiced with chili and local Alaea Red Sea salt, then placed in the centre of the green cradle. The flaps of the hanging leaves on the sides of the nest were tightly tugged around the filling. After securing the parcel with some wire, Alani wrapped the parcel once again in a few banana leaves and finally popped it on the hot coals to cook.

Then we all relaxed in the hammocks under the tree. Steven enlightened us about many kava mysteries, facts and legends, while Alani whipped up the sauce for the upcoming feast from pounded dried shrimp, a piece of fermented poi, chili powder, mango, salt and water.

As per Hawaiian folklore, the kava plant was brought to earth by twin gods – Kane and Kanaloa – who planted kava around the Hawaiian Islands and taught people about its use. In order to have good crops, kava farmers still pray to the gods and chant ritualistic poems. 'Awa was considered to be the staple food of the gods, which mortals had to use in order to get closer to them.

No religious ceremony is complete without 'awa, where it is offered to the gods in exchange for their blessing for success in marriage, health and fertility, a bountiful harvest or a good catch. This elaborate ceremonial ritual is very strict and detailed. It includes all procedures from making the kava libation, the ritual of spilling it on the ground and sprinkling it on the images of the gods and altar, to making the utensils such as the kanoa (kava cup), which is made from a polished coconut shell cut lengthwise.

Similar to the ambrosia of the ancient Greek gods, kava brew, with its psychoactive effects, is considered to be the only food of the Hawaiian gods, and is treated by the indigenous people with extreme respect.

Many Hawaiian legends describe conflicts and mischiefs between the gods fighting for the privilege of kava drinking. This found its way into the strictly observed practice by the locals around who could drink kava and when.

In approximately two hours, the sweet earthy aroma from the imu became very intense. The green juicy parcel was cleaned from the discoloured banana leaves and served on a large plate with sauce and thick fermented poi.

It looked like a simple dish – however, the combination of ingredients and the method of cooking turned it into a potent aphrodisiac. We thoroughly enjoyed the colourful dish known as laulau, with its intoxicating smoky-flavoured aroma and delicious morsels dipped in hot sauce, which perfectly complemented the multiple levels of tastes amalgamated in this dish.

The green leaves and the pink meat within the parcel were juicy and well cooked. The more we ate, the more we wanted to eat! However, we were not impressed by the starchy, purple-grey gooey poi, made from fermented taro root mash, with its sour smell, even though it happened to be most popular local side dish.

After the meal we tried Steven's own cloudy alcoholic aphrodisiac drink. Made with kava, lecithin emulsified water and the root of Hawaiian baby woodrose, it – along with the quantity of kava brew we consumed earlier – produced feelings of deep euphoria and sexual longing, attesting to Steven's affirmation of kava's aphrodisiac powers.

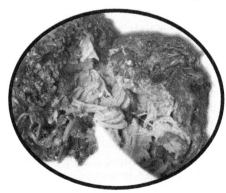

Steven's Cloudy Kava Recipe

100g kava root chopped
1 egg yolk (or 1 tablespoon of commercial lecithin)
1 ½ glasses of filtered or mineral water
100g Hawaiian baby woodrose root, dry
100g brown sugar
750ml white rum

Combine water, kava and woodrose roots and boil for ten minutes, then strain and let cool. Whisk egg yolk with brown sugar in separate bowl until sugar dissolves. Combine root extract with egg mixture, then vigorously whisk liquid, adding white rum slowly. Transfer into a jug. Serve with ice in tall glasses.

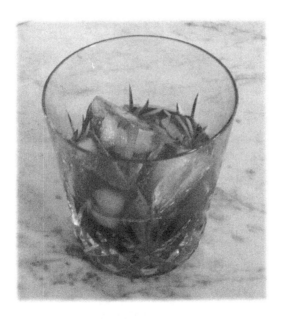

Legend: Oysters Casanova

Giacomo Casanova, the famous eighteenth-century lover and seducer, was known for his alluring charisma and insatiable hunger for love, which supposedly made him irresistible to women of all ages. However, not many know that he had a vital secret!

In his youth, Giacomo suffered from frequent nosebleeds and was successfully treated by the Witch of Venice, who also told the young man about the many rare herbs able to open women's hearts, and which later contributed to his life-long objective of seducing as many women as he could.

Parcels

>   12 oysters, fresh and large
>   12 spinach leaves, large
>   6 kava leaves

Sauce

>   100ml white wine
>   1 datura leaf
>   4 eggs yolks
>   2 tablespoons of cream, or coconut cream

Garnish

>   30ml brandy
>   ¼ lemon, zested
>   2 tablespoons of dill, chopped
>   12 asparagus tips, green, fresh
>   1 chili, fresh
>   Sea salt
>   1 baguette or crusty bread

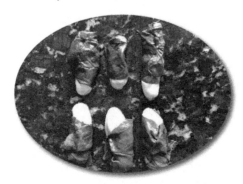

Many suspected this insatiable lover of witchcraft. He was even arrested and sentenced to five years imprisonment at the Piombi prison, from which he managed to escape. Here is one of his – allegedly – most famous recipes:

Open oysters using an oyster knife. Save the shells and the oyster liquid. Bring small pot of water to the boil. Place asparagus tips in a strainer and blanch them for a few seconds, before plunging into icy-cold water. Wrap each oyster in one spinach leaf, leaving the oyster's sexy naked tip to hang out.

In a wide saucepan, simmer white wine with chopped kava leaves. Gently immerse the wrapped oysters in the simmering wine and poach them for a minute. The oysters are ready when their naked ends are firm to the touch. Transfer oyster parcels back into the shells.

Combine the saved oyster liquid and finely chopped datura leaf to the remainder of the wine. Simmer for five minutes or until it's reduced by a third. Pour into a bowl, add cream, and whisk together adding, one by one, all the egg yolks until it's smooth. Slowly whisk the mixture into the simmering stock and immediately take off the heat. Add salt to taste and carefully pour one tablespoon of the sauce over each oyster.

Place a small bowl of freshly cut crusty bread and blanched asparagus in the centre of the plate. Place the oysters in their shells on the platter in a flower-like shape around the bowl. Add three drops of brandy to each oyster and decorate them with a mixture of chopped red chili, dill and lemon zest.

Casanova served this dish with a glass of bubbly and always insisted on feeding his lovers from his own hands … Voila! Enjoy your Oysters Casanova and … the delightful consequences!

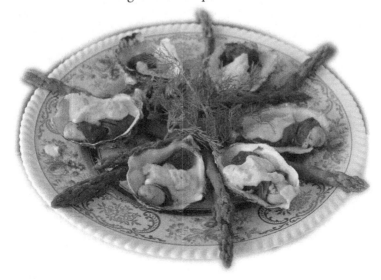

Deer Velvet – Japan

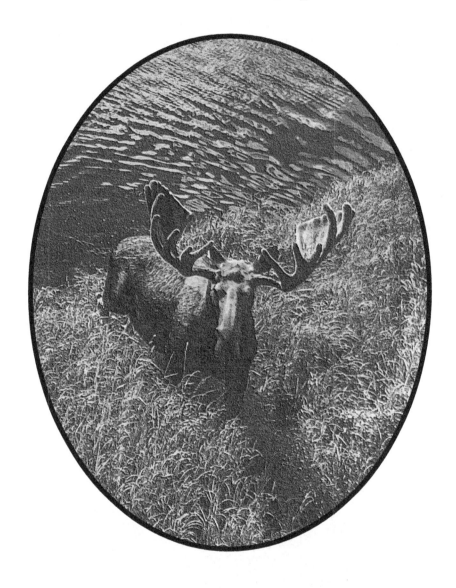

Antler horns contain excellent combination of calcium, phosphorus, magnesium, estrone, pantocrin, choline and other sterols, which proved to make overall revitalizing physical and mental effects for both sexes.

Dr. V.L.Zeltser

The unique cuisine of Japan seems to appeal to my senses. It's unusual cooking techniques and ingredients inevitably spark conversations between itamae (sushi chef) and me, forever curious about biyaku (aphrodisiacs in Japanese).

My collection of Japanese aphrodisiac recipes contains some old and unusual preparations of famous Kyoto geishas, elaborate treats of street vendors, and specially trained seafood chefs who prepare dangerous puffer fish sashimi. However in this chapter I would like to tell you about just one aphrodisiac – deer velvet.

Deer velvet is a velvet-like soft 'skin' that appears on the new antlers of deer, moose, elk and other members of the Cervidae species during mating season.

At a Japanese restaurant in Melbourne's CBD, I spoke to chef Haru, who mentioned that the most potent aphrodisiac (biyaku in Japanese) that he ever tried was soup made with deer velvet, which is very popular in Japan.

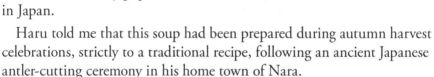

Haru told me that this soup had been prepared during autumn harvest celebrations, strictly to a traditional recipe, following an ancient Japanese antler-cutting ceremony in his home town of Nara.

He also said that the soup is more potent when made from fresh deer horns and is highly prized by the locals. With a naughty smile, Haru added that Japanese culture is known for many biyaku – however, he believed that deer horns outshone all other Japanese aphrodisiacs. Anecdotally, the Staghorn beetle, whose horns resemble deer antlers, are also sometimes made into soup, but more often are worn as sex amulets.

To my surprise, my husband confirmed that what Haru had told me might actually be true, as while he was studying medicine, he had came across the potent sex booster Pantocrine – an alcohol extract made from deer-antler velvet, which was available over the counter at pharmacies in Russia. Deer velvet is also known to stimulate production of human growth hormone, strengthen the immune system and bone density, and effectively assist in bodybuilding, which explains its ban from many sporting clubs and the World Anti-Doping Agency. My husband remembered experiencing euphoric prolonged orgasms after taking it.

I simply had to investigate this amazing aphrodisiac and experience its horny powers! After some persuasion I convinced my husband to travel that autumn to Nara to see this brutal ancient Japanese ritual, which happily co-exists alongside today's modern hi-tech lifestyle.

From Nara City Centre, we hopped on the public bus, which took us to the Rokuen Ceremony Arena, located in a vast picturesque and ecologically unspoiled park. There were many gorgeous spotted deer proudly wearing their huge antler crowns. They were smaller than their brothers – the large North American elks – but as courteous. Many of them were preoccupied with their lives, not paying any attention to the huge crowds of spectators.

I was probably a little too close to them, as our escort Akiyama-san quickly pointed out some damaged trees in the park. He warned us that they were used by the stags to sharpen their antlers and that it would be safer to keep a respectable distance from the aggressive stags during their mating season.

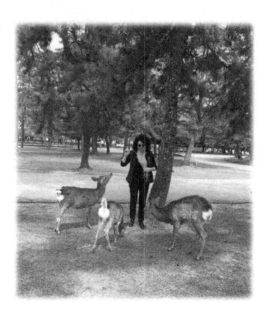

For this very reason, in 1671, Nara's magistrate established Shika no Tsunokiri – the Deer Antler-Cutting Ceremony – usually held over a three-day public holiday at a specially assembled place – the Rokuen arena – at the Kofukuji Temple. In reality, this 30-minute ceremony is a kind of Japanese deer rodeo or corrida (bullfight), where sacred deer are blessed by the priests and 'lock horns' with specially trained men, in a theatrical battle of man against beast!

After a traditional prayer, the first group of bucks were let into the arena, where men armed with red flags pushed them towards two seko (deer herdsman), who attempted to lasso them with juji (a hand-held wooden device attached to the long rope).

When caught, one by one, the bucks were secured to the wooden posts in the middle of the arena and forced to lie down. The excited crowd listened with rapt attention to the commentator over the loud speaker, accompanied by the drum tremolo. After that, six men carried a buck to the ceremonial blanket, and held down its head on the pillow for the cutting procedure.

The main priest of the temple – the shinkan – comforted the scared animal by patting it with his white gloves and giving it some water. Then, accompanied by the rhythmic drum beats, he quickly sawed off its antlers with a sawblade and released the buck, unsuspecting of its loss, back into the park, leaving behind the highly prized antlers as an offering to the god of the Kasuga Shrine.

This ancient ceremony somehow reminded me of the bulls that I've seen killed by matadors at the Spanish corrida.

I couldn't help but feel sorry for the deer's loss, but I was happy to see them freed without the loss of any other body parts, knowing that in Chinese Medicine, the tails, meat, testicles and especially the penis are believed to increase lust very effectively and as such are highly valued. Even bezoar – deer gall stones – are highly prized in folk medicine and some shamanic traditions as an antivenin and powerful sexual stimulant.

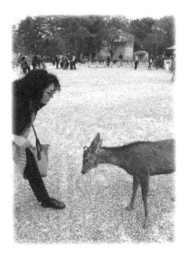

Later that day we were introduced to the local deer-antler trader Riku-san, whose family had been involved in the business for almost 500 years. He was slim and well over eighty years of age, with a thick main of slightly grey hair on his head and straight posture. He was obviously sexually active, as he – perhaps deliberately! – cast some hot looks my way, which made me blush. Weird!

With few words, he invited us into his cosy showroom to see his display of deer velvet, from the antlers of the hormone-charged spotted sika stag. There were tons of other deer-antler products: frozen, dried, whole, thinly sliced in discs, crushed, pulverised, made into tinctures, alcoholic extracts and tea mixtures, as well as books containing recipes, deer skins, horn-cutting gadgets, dried deer penises, deer images, pungent sprays and soaps, and more.

Riku-san pointed out that his main customers were tourists, which proves that the use of deer horns as an aphrodisiac wasn't specific only to the Japanese culture.

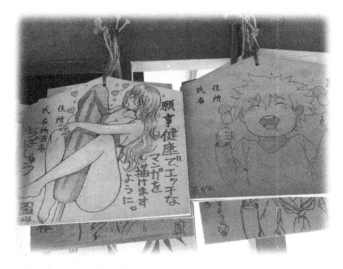

Thousands of years ago, wherever deer freely roamed in the wild, people managed to link the appearance of the deer's crown during mating season to an increase in their sexual vigour. Thinking that this could be passed on to humans, they identified it as an aphrodisiac – and one still highly prized for its unique chemical composition able to increase sexual drive and sperm count.

I remembered spotting frozen deer horns at the farmers markets in Banff in Canada and health shops in New Zealand. It seems that every nation has its own unique rituals, customs and recipes for tinctures, love potions, soups, sniffing powders, teas and alcoholic brews, incense and amulets. Deer horns also decorate the walls in many different countries as a symbol of masculinity and sexual strength.

It is strange that the term 'wearing horns' refers to a man being a cuckold instead of being sexually charged. Perhaps it actually refers to a man being defeated by a stronger male? In fact, it actually alludes to the mating habits of stags, who forfeit their mates when they are defeated by another male.

Riku-san was also aware of Pantocrine, which he used to import from Russia – however, it had become too expensive, so instead he offered us his potent bōru (deer balls). Deer balls? Seeing my disgusted facial expression, the shopkeeper invited us to see how the potent deer balls were made.

All ingredients for the secret recipe were measured and placed into a ceramic bowl. Then they were were continuously mixed for at least fifteen to twenty minutes. Riku-san would stop occasionally to smell the mixture until it became homogenous and gained the strength that the old trader wanted. Finally Riku-san invited us to help him shape the mass into hazelnut-sized balls. With fingertips dipped in sesame oil to prevent sticking, we made many balls, which were dropped into a bag with cocoa powder for coating. Then each ball was placed into an individual paper cup and stacked into a specially designed lacquered box.

The balls had a pleasant slightly gamey aroma and tangy citrusy flavour, mixed with the scent of dark chocolate. The trader warned us that the balls were very potent and known to produce a valuable cumulative effect if taken every day before breakfast on an empty stomach, and that two balls a day was the maximum adult dosage. Then he packed those balls and gave them to us as a gift.

I have to admit, that after only two of these 'balls', my husband and I were both absolutely smitten by their immediate impact on our libido.

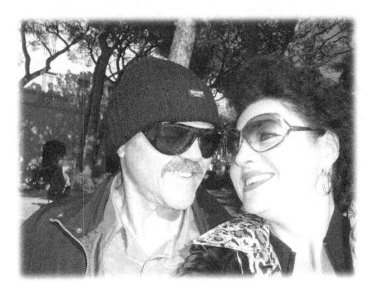

67

Riku-san's Horny Balls

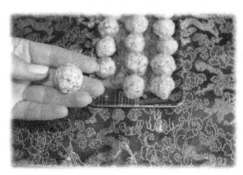

100g deer velvet powder
100g fermented soybean powder
100g gingko biloba nuts, crushed and roasted
100g cold-pressed honey
50g cocoa powder (or almond flour, poppy seeds or toasted sesame seeds)
30g orange blossoms, dried and rubbed

Mix all ingredients, with the exception of the honey, into sticky dough for ten minutes using an electric mixer. Dip fingers into sesame oil and shape dough into hazelnut-sized balls. Drop balls into a plastic bag filled with a few spoons of cocoa powder. Gently shake bag and lay out dusted balls in an air-tight container. Keep in a dark, cool place.

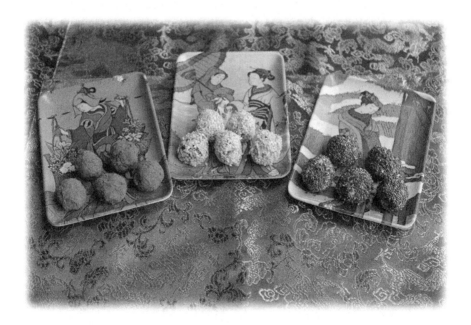

Horny Rolls

This splendid recipe was given to me by Kim Bae, who hosted our ginseng expedition to Korea. It's called Mallin Gotgamssam – dried persimmons stuffed with a filling made similarly to Riku-san's deer balls. Over the years, this colourful and highly potent recipe has earned me lots of compliments.

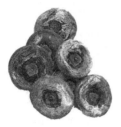

4 persimmons, dried
30g deer velvet powder
50g apricots, dried and minced
16 halved walnuts
2 tablespoons of cold-pressed honey

Mix water, honey, powdered deer velvet and minced apricots into a soft dough. Leave mixture to stand in a cool place for ten to fifteen minutes. With a sharp knife, cut off the persimmon leaves and make an incision in the middle, leaving the other side of the persimmon uncut. Unfold, and flatten persimmon with your fingers, remove any seeds and trim to create a rectangular shape. Spread two rectangles on plastic wrap side by side and evenly cover with filling. Place walnut halves in the centre as if recreating whole walnuts. Using the wrap, gently roll the persimmon, taking care that the filling and nuts are covered.

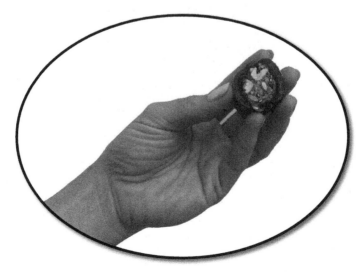

Twist the ends of the plastic wrap, compress into a firm roll and place into the freezer for at least twenty minutes.

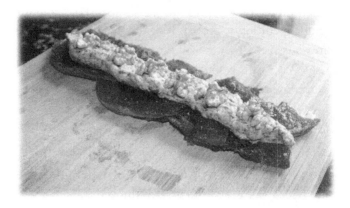

Unwrap and cut with a sharp knife into slices resembling sliced deer antlers. Serve as a dessert or snack. This easy-to-make potent aphrodisiac snack can be frozen for up to three months.

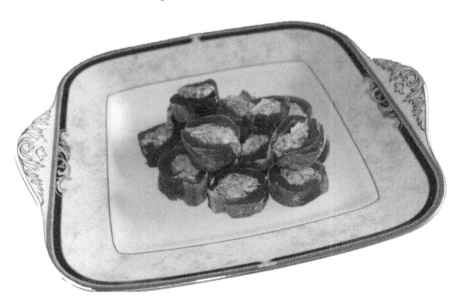

Legend: Size Matters

Not many have heard the true story of how Tsar Peter the Great met his wife Catherine I, the first Empress of Russia.

Tsar Peter was indeed a 'great' Russian tsar, remembered for his extensive reforms which saw Russia established as a great nation. For his achievements and his giant physique – at nearly seven feet tall – he was nick-named Peter the Great. However, due to these great proportions, the Tsar faced a challenge in finding women suitable for his physical magnitude! His first wife could not bear his 'greatness' for too long and hid herself in the monastery. The news about his dilemma travelled fast and soon everyone knew the Russian tsar was looking for a new wife!

Miles away in a provincial Swedish town, there lived a young peasant girl of generous proportions named Martha, who also had a problem finding the right man to marry. When she heard about the Tsar's dilemma, she decided to test her luck, walking all the way to St Petersburg where she was employed to work in the kitchen of the Tsar's best friend – Prince Alexander Menshikov. Her exceptional features soon got her into the prince's bed. However, when Alexander was lost in her grand-size delights, he decided to use his discovery as an opportunity to strengthen his friendship with the Tsar.

Realising that kitchen-maid Martha would not attract Peter, he invited the Tsar to his palace for dinner. However, before that he bought an aphrodisiac from the local alchemist and ordered his chef to secretly add it to the Tsar's food. He also arranged for Martha to be the only female table-servant.

Everything went according to plan. When the Tsar's sexual desire was on fire beyond any control, he advanced himself to the most-welcoming Martha … and the aphrodisiac obviously worked.

For the first time in their lives, both lovers experienced diamonds in the sky. Tsar Peter the Great married Martha, who eventually was crowned as Catherine I – the first Empress of Russia – who never forgot Prince Alexander Menshikov's endeavour.

Recipe:
Brew

50g thinly sliced deer antlers
400ml vodka
150ml water

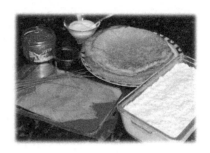

Blini (crepes)
½ cup white flour
¼ teaspoon of baking soda
1 tablespoon of vegetable oil
½ teaspoon of sea salt
1 large egg, lightly beaten
1 cup cold milk or water
40g salted butter
1 soft-boiled egg
3 tablespoons of red (salmon) caviar
3 tablespoons of black (osetra) caviar
½ cup crème fraîche or sour cream
8 thin slices of fresh salmon fillet
4 fresh oysters

Garnish

1 bunch of chives, finely chopped
1 bunch of dill, finely chopped
4 asparagus spears

Place sliced deer antlers into a small pot. Cover with 150 ml of cold water, and bring to boil. Reduce heat, cover with lid, and simmer for thirty minutes. Strain the brew and let it cool down to the room temperature.

Peel and mash soft-boiled egg, add chopped dill, salt and black pepper to taste, then mix with two tablespoons of the brew. Smudge this spread on the thinly sliced salmon, cover and place in the fridge.

Mix the rest of the deer velvet brew with vodka and place it in the fridge.

Whisk fresh egg with sea salt into a foam; keep on mixing while adding bi-carbonated soda, milk or water, oil and flour. Let the batter stand for ten minutes. Pre-heat pancake pan and make eight large thin blini. Spread butter on each blin (crepe) while they are still hot, stack and keep warm.

Mix crème fraîche with chives and divide into eight portions. Place each portion in the centre of each blin, top it up with a teaspoon of salmon caviar and roll it into a tube. Fold tubes in half, and slightly cut open at the middle exposing the red caviar. Using two tubes, form an ellipsoid shape on the serving plate. Line ellipsoid with marinated salmon, and place beluga caviar around the edge of the ellipsoid. Position an oyster at the inner top corner of the ellipsoid. Blanch asparagus, dip tips in cold brew and place in the centre of the composition. Scatter some left-over dill and chopped chives on the outer rim of each plate. Serve immediately with icy-cold brew. The suggestive presentation of this dish contributes to the sensual arousal and enhancement of the experience. Enjoy the pleasant, lasting effect of the royal treat and its consequences!

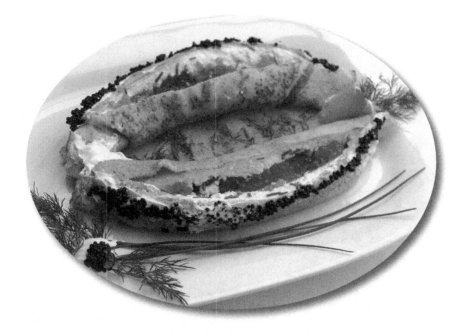

Yohimbe – Cameroon

Pausinystalia johimbe (Latin), locally known as Love Tree Pausinystalia

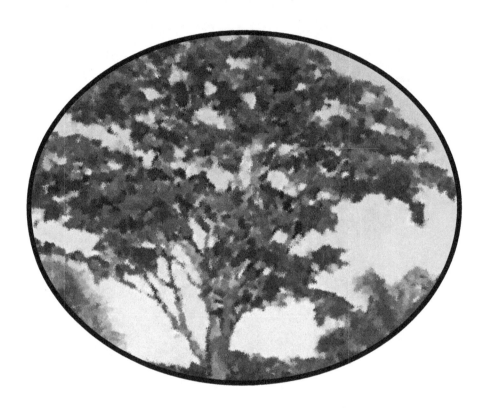

This plant contains unique alkaloids, that dilate small arteries by blocking the release of neurotransmitters, which regulate blood flow to sex organs through their impact on the arteries. It is known to produce strong erection in males and heightened sensual pleasure, however it is also known for its unpleasant toxic side effects like nausea, irritability, and excessive perspiration. Dr. V.L.Zeltser

This Central African aphrodisiac adventure was, strangely, instigated by a cup of coffee I ordered at a small coffee shop in Melbourne's CBD. As I looked at the young, handsome barista Paul, I playfully said that I felt like an aphrodisiac fix. He smiled with his plump lips and politely said that he grew up in Cameroon on a coffee plantation and that coffee was not really an aphrodisiac! However, in his village, many people use yohimbe tree, known in Cameroon as 'love tree', to enhance sex and libido.

I undertook some research, which proved the barista to be correct. For thousands of years before viagra was developed, the unique aphrodisiac qualities of yohimbe were known and used by African tribes. In the eighteenth century, it was brought to Europe by merchants as a magic sexual stimulant, where it gained instant popularity as an aphrodisiac, fetching high prices.

Even now this highly effective aphrodisiac competes head to head with the pharmaceutical giants, which have caused it to be banned in some countries. However, due to public demand, it always finds its way back.

We started planning our next trip to Cameroon to hunt for this African aphrodisiac in its natural habitat.

As per advice received from the Mbalmayo National Forestry School, we headed to Mbalmayo city, which is located near Cameroon's oldest forest reserve – home of practically every variety of flora and fauna found in tropical Africa. Friendly local botanist Joseph assisted us on our quest.

An experienced forager armed with a sharp machete, Joseph guided our hunt through the magnificent evergreen backwoods of this local forest, where yohimbe trees still grow in the wild. Pointing at the scars on the bark of some of the trees, Joseph explained that these were the signs of them having been harvested before.

There were many yohimbe trees around us. Joseph told us that locals compare yohimbe trees to African men. They are slim, strong, tall and persuasive and can make women feel very happy!

Soon I could easily recognise yohimbe trees, as they stood out in the wilderness of the forest among the palm trees – their branches full of juicy, pointy oval-shaped leaves and 'clever' small seeds hiding in the paper-thin winged slivers. Attractive trees indeed!

The hallucinogenic, libido-enhancing qualities of the yohimbe tree have been known to indigenous African tribes for thousands of years, who have used yohimbe in sacred amok rituals, as well as for poisoning hunting arrows, to treat frigidity and impotence, increase fertility, and to induce deep orgasms.

When the potent chemical yohimbine was discovered by Western pharmacology in the pinkish-brown bark and the yellow heartwood of the trunk of yohimbe trees, its bark became highly profitable for the locals. Using rotating bark-harvesting techniques, local villagers protect the trees from plant pirates, who cut them down and cause overharvesting.

With a few powerful movements Joseph quickly cut off a diamond-shaped piece of bark with his sharp machete and peeled it off the trunk without harming the sacrosanct native tree. It seemed easy to do, and soon each of us collected a sample of approximately ten by twenty centimetres of the moist bark with its woody smell.

All Joseph's friends used yohimbe bark on a regular basis, as it was believed to be harmless and yet highly beneficial for general health, strength of muscles, and – most importantly – increasing the size and sensitivity of the genitals through massive surges of blood flow.

Stopping by a large shrub and with a happy chuckle, Joseph introduced it as khat (Catha edulis) – another African aphrodisiac plant! For centuries, this plant has stimulated libido and improved the mood of the native tribes. I picked up some of the leaves, and we chewed them for the rest of our journey, feeling content and stimulated as if we had drunk a few strong coffees.

However, by late afternoon I felt totally exhausted by the hot sticky weather and could not wait to get back to my air-conditioned hotel room, bypassing Joseph's offer to demonstrate the ancient Cameroon technique of yohimbe bark preparation.

Joseph decided to help me by offering a cigar, which he rolled using a mix of yohimbe bark specks, mixed with tobacco. It was too hot to smoke, however Joseph assured me that the cigar would make me perspire and cool down, and that they were harmless and commonly used by the locals to combat fatigue.

It was a local gesture of friendship, traditionally practised by the natives to help each other with the hard work of harvesting yohimbe bark from the mature trees at the yohimbe farms during rainy seasons, when it has the greatest alkaloid content.

It wasn't polite for me to reject Joseph's psychoactive treat, and to my surprise, I soon felt a sudden surge of energy in my limbs and became more tolerant to the heat due to the cooling evoporation of my sweat.

At Joseph's house, we washed our samples, shredded them into small pieces and placed one handful into the pot. After pouring some boiling water over it, the yohimbe bark was left to brew for ten to fifteen minutes. Finally, the amber liquid was strained into another pot, to which Joseph added few slices of lemon, honey and a teaspoon of cinnamon bark powder.

After delicious tribal dinner we drank this sweet and sour muddy concoction, anxious to experience yohimbe magic. However, while it was obvious that it made Joseph feel amazing, the brew did not seem to produce any aphrodisiac effect on my husband or me, other than a headache. Surprised, Joseph suggested that it was probably due to the level of excitement that we had experienced that day, and perhaps it would kick in later. Well, he was right!

That night, the full magic of yohimbe's powers was revealed, and in the morning, we felt like newlyweds. Thank you, Joseph, for this unforgettable experience which made it well worth our while going all the way to Africa!

Back home, my husband researched and explained the phenomenon we had experienced: yohimbine is the indole alkaloid of the yohimbe tree bark, which is known to have an accumulative effect. This allows regular users to feel its effects immediately, while first-time users usually experience a delayed reaction. Yohimbe is known to increase the level of norepinephrine, a neurotransmitter in the brain, which is carried by the bloodstream to the adrenal glands, and as a result, it causes an increase in energy, stress endurance, physical performance and heightened sexuality.

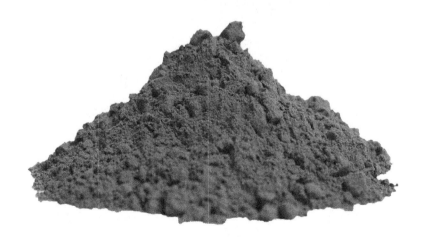

Joseph's Recipe

1 litre of water
6 teaspoons yohimbe bark, grinded or finely chipped
1 teaspoon of cinnamon bark powder (or vanilla extract)
½ lemon
3 tablespoons of cold-pressed honey (optional)

Bring to boil 1 litre of water (I used still mineral water with a high alkaloids count). Add yohimbe bark to boiled water, and brew for ten to fifteen minutes. Strain, then add cinnamon bark powder or vanilla extract, lemon – which makes the brew soluble and aromatic – and honey to taste, if you wish. Drink slowly, relax and experience the delightful effects.

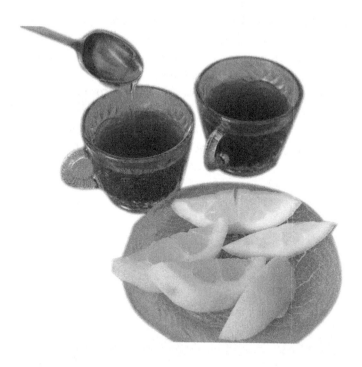

Legend: Love & War

In eighteenth-century France, adultery was a perfectly acceptable social phenomenon – in fact, lovers were looked at as marriage saviours, rather than marriage destroyers. However, jealous Italian-born Napoleon Bonaparte couldn't bear the thought of sharing his forever-hungry-for-love Josephine with anyone, despite the fact that his potency greatly suffered from the stress, and physical and mental exhaustion of his on-going war campaigns.

Desperate Napoleon secretly consulted alchemists, botanists and physicians in France and in all the countries he conquered, until one day, he learned about the miraculous African potency tree, or yohimbe, which guaranteed men to be ready at any time with an enlarged penis. It was also said to strengthen stamina and lengthen the pleasure of the sexual act. The tree grew in the wilderness of Africa, and was accessible only through the spice traders of faraway Egypt, who sold this wonder aphrodisiac for its weight in gold.

Determined to keep his wife happy without the help of lovers, Napoleon assured his government of an easy victory over the Ottoman territories of Egypt and Syria, and ventured into Africa, where he quickly learned how to brew the magic potion from the bark of the yohimbe tree.

Happy with the effects of the aphrodisiac, for weeks Napoleon indulged in sensual pleasures with Josephine in their gold and blue silk tent, while his heat-exhausted soldiers continued to lose battles.

When he became aware of the poor situation of his army, Napoleon ordered yohimbe bark to be confiscated from all spice merchants and mixed into his soldiers daily red wine ration. The magic worked! The testosterone-charged soldiers fought much harder for their wives at home alone and their beloved leader. They conquered Africa and most of the European Continent, extending French control into Asia, which gave Napoleon a reason to proclaim himself as emperor. And so it was, this humble African aphrodisiac helped Napoleon gain much more than he bargained for!

Recipe:

300g yohimbe bark powder
750ml red wine or other alcohol with min 13% alc/vol
250ml filtered water
3 tablespoons of cold-pressed honey
12 cloves

Place powdered yohimbe bark and cloves in a small pot. Cover with water and simmer for fifteen to twenty minutes, occasionally stirring, until two-thirds of the water has evaporated. Add a glass of red wine and let brew for ten minutes. Strain liquid and combine with the remaining wine, add honey to taste, and transfer liquid into a dark glass bottle with air-tight cap.

A single shot glass of this drink managed to produce two plus hours of unforgettable sensual indulgence and euphoria for my husband and I!

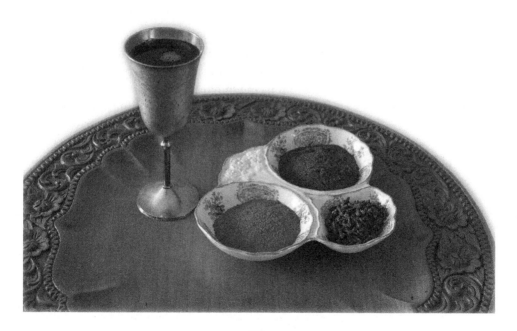

Horny Goat Weed – China

Epimedium or Yin Yang Huo, also known as Bishop's Hat, Fairy Wings and Barrenwort

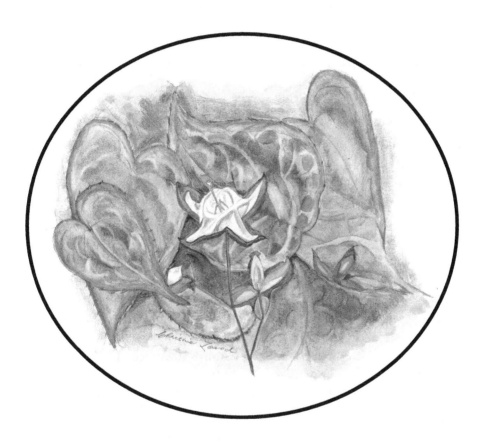

This plant contains unique fusion of vitamin E , icariin, benzene, tannin, sterols, and palmitic and linoleic acids, which can help men to balance hormones, rise sperm count and semen density, and improve blood flow to the penis.   *Dr. V.L.Zeltser*

One day when my dear friend Xin Chen Yong and I were enjoying some afternoon tea in my garden, she picked a few leaves from my elf dwarf tree and added them to the teapot, saying that they looked exactly like the leaves of the aphrodisiac herb, horny goat weed, or yin yang huo in Chinese. When she was twelve, she used to go to the mountains with her aunt Phoung to forage for this herb, as it was prescribed by the local herbalist to her childless uncle Li.

A few years later, Xin migrated to Australia and heard that her fifty-seven-year-old uncle Li had fathered two children with his forty-nine-year-old wife, after not having been able to conceive for twenty-five years.

My husband's quick research confirmed that Chinese herbal medicine recognises yin yang huo as a remedy for barrenness and an aphrodisiac, as it dilates the corpora cavernosa, which channels blood to the penis, facilitating erection.

More so, this particular aphrodisiac is known to accumulate its stimulating properties in the human body, revitalising and stabilising the natural sexual response, which is more than can be said for many pharmaceuticals that mechanically force erection for a short period of time.

Unsurprisingly, this discovery fuelled my interest to experience horny goat weed – which led us to its birthplace, China.

As in many other countries I have visited, it wasn't easy to get the locals to talk about aphrodisiacs, due to the fact that – despite their global popularity – sexual stimulants are often tabooed due to the level of education, personal reasons, culture, religion, and clouds of unknown and uncertain information spread by pharmaceutical companies in an attempt to protect their markets.

That's where we really appreciated the help of Xin's uncle. With the help of Google Translate, the now seventy-eight-year-old Li managed to arrange a meeting for us with his herbalist Dr Ling and a few local foragers.

We met with Dr Ling at his herbal medicine practice of forty years. A knowledgeable herbalist, Dr Ling told us that horny goat weed is a pharmacologically certifiable herb with potent active ingredients which enhance sexual excitement and responsiveness, memory and brain capacity, by promoting better blood flow and circulation. Within days, male patients usually experience potency revival due to the rise of semen production, while women experience an increase in sexuality and genital sensitivity.

For these reasons, many herbalists often use horny goat weed in combination with other herbs and substances beneficial to health in the famous 'Spring Wine' – a Taoist's miracle equivalent to the European 'Elixir of Life' – where it is combined with other aphrodisiacs such as ginseng, deer velvet resin, red lizard, wolfberry, angelica root and other botanicals, and steeped in rice wine for a month.

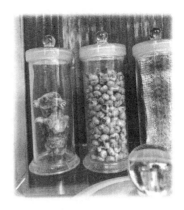

With a strange grin, Dr Ling offered us the chance to experience the power of horny goat weed and asked his shop assistant to brew it for us at the back of the shop. It arrived in tulip-shaped ceramic cups – an amber-coloured liquid with a grassy aroma and surprisingly pleasant, slightly bitter-sweet taste.

After the first few sips I could feel a distinctive warmth travel from my abdomen to my head, then to my limbs and other parts of my body. This unexpectedly pleasant sensation lasted for an hour or so. Later that day, I brewed the same bitter-sweet drink using Dr Ling's recipe, however it produced a rather lesser effect compared to the one we experienced at his shop.

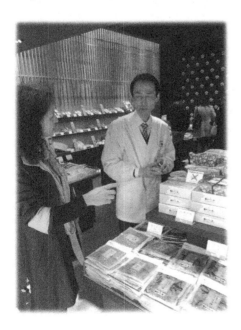

I went to see Dr Ling again to clarify where I had gone wrong and why we were missing out on the delicious feelings we had experienced at the shop. However Dr Ling was out, and his assistant explained that horny goat weed, being an adaptogen, produces a preview of what it can do when it is used for the first time. However, with regular use, it accumulates in the body, effectively stabilising sexual drive. His advice proved to be correct.

Next day Uncle Li and middle-aged foragers Evan and

his wife Sha walked us to the nearby mountain forest to search for horny goat weed plants in the wild. Evan, who had been foraging for herbs in these mountains for their shop in town for the last twenty years, easily found a patch of horny goat weed, which happily grew on the forest floor of the moist humus-rich soil.

We collected three bagfuls of the leaves and one bag of intricate horny goat weed flowers, which varied in colour and had a distinct four-part layered structure, with light-green outer sepals, followed by a few more layers of large brightly coloured inner petals. Sha told me that locals use

them to make popular 'love pillows', which induce a desirable deep sleep filled with sweet sexual dreams. For that, the flowers need to be sun-dried and then mixed with another wonder plant – motherwort – and stuffed into the silk pillow case.

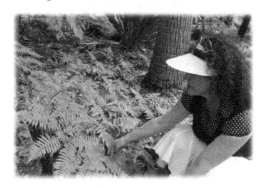

The fresh mountain air made us hungry and I was happy when Evan and Sha invited us to try some local horny goat delicacies, which they intended to cook in the forest. As if by magic, all the necessary utensils, ingredients and even a tiny portable gas burner came out from Evan's rucksack. Sitting on the rocks, warmed from the sun, armed with chopsticks and plastic spoons, we enjoyed Evan's tasty aphrodisiacs – hot tea from his thermos (similar in taste to Dr Ling's tea) and a green mouth-watering prawn casserole, prepared by Sha.

According to local legend, over 2,000 years ago an old shepherd named Huo took his goats to this mountain to graze. The goats ate some plants with heart-shaped green leaves after which they became friskier and more sexually active. The shepherd decided to try this herb too, and he experienced a similar effect despite his old age.

He collected plants and brought them to the temple in his village, where they were distributed to willing villagers. Since that time, the fame of the horny goat weed has spread all over China for its ability to stimulate libido, restore sexual energy, treat impotence, enhance sexual desire and libido, and increase production of semen in men, as well as to treat suppressed libido in women due to menopause.

After the picnic, my husband and I felt distinctly arousing sexual pulsations in our genitals, which continued for a few hours. Since Sha cooked very quickly, I could not record any details of her recipe. However, on our return home, with the help of my friend Xin, I recreated this recipe, which admittedly tasted and worked almost as well as the original, inducing in us playful behaviour, lustfulness and sexual urges.

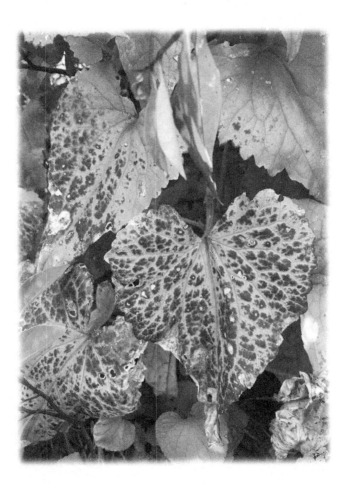

Horny Goat Weed & Prawns

300g horny goat weed leaves, fresh or 50g dried
2 tablespoons of sesame oil
2 tablespoons of fermented shrimp paste
1 bundle of ong choy (water spinach), trimmed and washed
3 cloves of garlic, crushed
12 large peeled prawns (frozen prawns work as well)
Pack of flat rice noodles (I use fresh noodles from the Chinese grocer)

Serves 5

Prepare flat rice noodles as per instructions on the pack. Heat up skillet, add sesame oil, then shrimp paste and crushed garlic. Stir for one minute, and then add horny goat weed leaves. Cover lid and let cook for two minutes. Stir in ong choy and add prawn. Cover and let prawns cook for about two minutes on each side, till they become baby pink. Serve hot over flat rice noodles. Add fresh chili and soy sauce to taste.

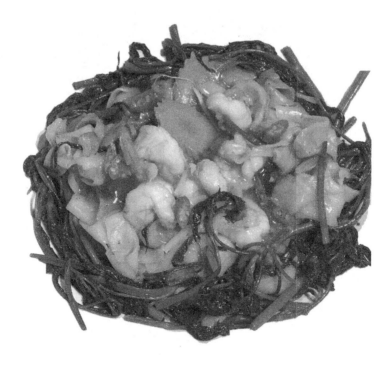

Dr Ling's Horny Goat Weed Tea & Liqueur

The following two recipes were kindly provided by Dr Ling. Both, tea and alcohol tincture (liqueur), contain natural soluble essential oils and minerals, and are equally effective.

Tea:

Add 40g of dried leaves or 20g of horny goat weed powder into a tea pot with 400ml of boiling water, stir, and allow to brew for ten minutes. Add cold-pressed honey to taste. Drink slowly on an empty stomach to enhance its effectiveness. This tea can be enjoyed up to three times a day.

Liqueur:

Place 225g of fresh horny goat weed leaves (or 70g dried) into a glass jar, add 750ml of any alcohol of your preference, close the lid and shake the jar for one to two minutes. Place in a cool dry cabinet of your kitchen or cellar, and let it infuse till the liqueur is a light caramel colour. Strain liquid and discard the leaves, if you do not wish to use them.

Over the years I have made this liqueur with red wine, vodka and whisky, with the last being my husband's favourite. The recommended dose is subject to your herbalist's advice, which can range from 20 to 50 ml of extract per day.

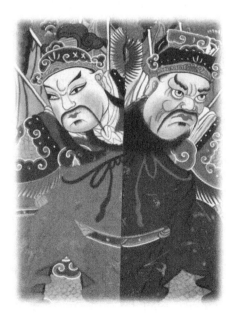

Legend: *Arabian Nights*

Who has not heard of the famous erotic Persian tales of 1001 nights? Did you really think that the powerful middle-aged Shahriyar, the ruler of the great Persian Empire, was interested in listening to Scheherazade's stories for 1001 nights instead of having hot sex? Or that his first wife had lost her mind when she committed adultery with the black cook, causing Shahriyar to become vindictive towards all women and kill his new virgin wives after the first night they spent together?

The truth is that when there were no more virgins left in the kingdom to marry, the witty Scheherazade, who was a little more experienced in love matters than was expected, was offered to him as a wife. Thus, during their first night together, she discovered Shahriyar's shameful secret – impotence, and had to resort to the only thing that could save her life – revival of his libido with the 'hush-hush' potion known to be used in the harems of Arabia. It was made from the expensive herbs – horny goat weed and khat, imported by the Silk Road merchants from China and Africa.

Clever Scheherazade managed to convince Shahriyar to hear her story before he sent her to the gallows by telling him that a jinnee had appeared to her before their wedding, and told her that she was destined to deliver a cure to her husband by telling him the following story:

'Once upon a time in the wilderness of the mountain forest of Northern China, there lived ferocious beasts with tremendous stamina and very strong sexual appetite. The beasts were known have sex up to a hundred times a day with anyone they could find. The emperor, who had many beautiful wives, became very jealous of the beasts and sent his spies to find out their secret.

'After a few days, his sneaky spies came back with piles of green leaves, which the beasts ate plenty of. The emperor's old herbalist turned this find into a delicious potent liqueur and named it Hush-Hush. Regretfully his attempt to personally test the potion before giving it to the emperor led him to jail for his sexual advances towards the emperor's wives. However, the recipe worked, and soon the emperor's sexual desire was on fire. He kept all his wives happy and managed to father a hundred children in one year. Then he pardoned his alchemist and gave him three beautiful maidens as a gift. Would you like me to make it for you, my Padishah?'

The curious man decided to try it … and, as the story goes, after 1001 nights, stimulated by Scheherazade's erotic stories, her beauty and potent aphrodisiac potion, Shahriyar fathered many children and they lived happily ever after.

Recipe:
2 tablespoons of cold-pressed honey
70g horny goat weed leaves, dried
10g khat leaves, dried
2 pieces of ginseng root, 2-3 cm each
1 teaspoon of fresh ginger, grated
50g cilantro (coriander) seeds, crushed
½ lemon, zested
1 bottle of red wine, brandy (or purified water, if you do not wish to use alcohol)

Gently rub dried horny goat weed and khat leaves in your palms, then place the flakes into a jar. Add ginseng roots, grated ginger, powdered cilantro seeds, honey and lemon zest, and top up jar with your preferred liquid (wine, brandy or water). Seal the jar and shake well until the honey is totally dissolved.

Place it on the windowsill or somewhere else with plenty of direct sunlight for three days. Twice a day, gently shake the jar. On the fourth day, drain the liquid through muslin cloth into a dark glass bottle and close with an air-tight cap. Keep sealed bottle in a cold, dark place (fridge or cellar).

Please note that water-based Hush-Hush needs to be kept in the fridge at all times and used within five days.

Take one teaspoon every morning before breakfast and a 30ml shot before bed. Enjoy the heightened sensuality and euphoria of sexual bliss.

This remedy works through the build-up of certain elements in the body – thus the speed and efficiency of the process depends on the health of the user!

Ashwagandha – Nepal

Withania somniferan ('sleep-inducing' in Latin)
Indian Ginseng or Winter Cherry

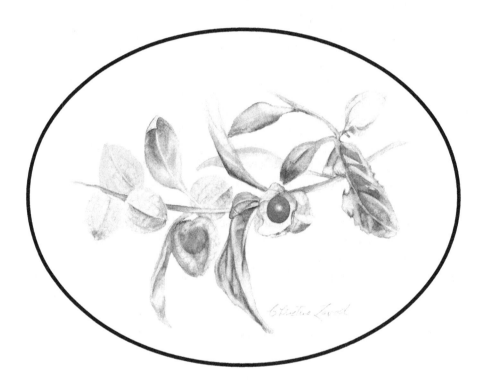

This nontoxic plant contains numerous nutrients, including plant sterols,
which are known to increase muscle mass, vitality and promote sexual
responsiveness.   *Dr. V.L.Zeltser*

Many years ago, when we ordered a bottle of chilled Italian white at a café on the Piazza della Signoria overlooking Florence's famous sculptural collections, the wine came served wvith six pieces of exotic fruit. Each looked like an elaborate paper-thin lantern with one bright-orange tomato-size berry inside, which – like the beautiful women of a harem – were hiding from the world behind dry, papery husks! Encouraged by our waiter, I squashed one berry in my mouth. It was loaded with slippery seeds, similar to tomato seeds, but with an unusual tart taste and sweet hints of pineapple and mango. Happy with me sampling this treat, the waiter explained that it was a new fruit called 'golden berries' or 'love gooseberries', which were known as a Peruvian aphrodisiac imported from South America. I was intrigued … However, after eating all six of them and not feeling any aphrodisiac effects, the berries were soon forgotten, until a decade later when I came across a similar-looking berry in Tibet, while on an expedition exploring the native aphrodisiac plant, ashwagandha.

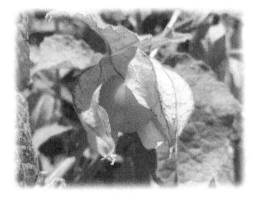

When we arrived in Jyamrung village, we were greeted with the peaceful sounds of cattle and twinkling chimes, birds and roosters. The village was surrounded by picturesque terrace fields nestled in the lush green landscape of the impressive Himalayan Mountains. The high altitude air was filled with the aromas of flowers, dried grass, snow and a little smoke.

Our friendly host Ballabh was a local middle-aged farmer, who spoke a little English he had picked up working in hotels before his marriage, and who we were lucky enough to meet.

We stayed for two days at his simple cosy house with million-dollar views of the mountain peaks. It felt like stepping a few centuries back in time, when different values were in place and life was full of simple pleasures and sensuality. We ate only homemade organic food, like yak-milk cheese, delicious hemp and wheat bread, local honey and candied fruit, as well as drinking plenty of green tea and traditional Nepalese bhang (a mixture of buffalo milk, hemp blossoms, datura seeds, cardamom, cinamon and honey).

While Ballabh was hosting us, his wife and kids were busy working in the nearby fields singing in Nepalese about their favourite hemp plant being a gift from Shiva – the Supreme Being who creates, protects and transforms the universe.

When we were ready to explore the wilderness, Ballabh explained that, unfortunately now, at the end of August, it would be very difficult to spot any ashwagandha shrubs in the wild, as the small shrubs were usually eaten up by native animals. Besides, there was no real advantage in looking for wild plants as the farmed ashwagandha here was as organic as the wild version.

The farmers do not use pesticides or fertilisers as they simply cannot afford them, thus the plants are grown commercially in an ecologically clean, natural environment. Local authorities encourage villagers to grow ashwagandha and other medicinal herbs as their high returns provide support to the Nepalese economy.

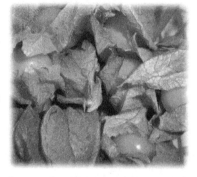

We climbed to one of the field terraces, decorated with colourful garlands of wind-ragged prayer flags and piles of small bright-orange fruit drying under the sun on the straw mats spread on the ground. Ashwagandha seedlings are planted in early spring and harvested in late summer, hence the local name – 'summer berries'. After the ashwagandha plants are harvested, the berries are usually left behind to sun-dry on the mats.

Ballabh picked a few ashwagandha lanterns from the small bush nearby and easily popped out the red berries with his thumb and offered them to me. They tasted similar to the ones I had tried years ago in

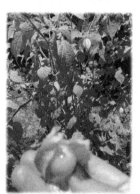

Florence and also in Peru, where they were known as 'Incan berries' or 'Pichu-berries'. The taste was like a mix of unripened cherry tomatoes and mango, however the same fruit semidried on the nearby mats had a more intense, sweet taste similar to sun-dried cherry tomatoes.

Ballabh explained that the dried berries are traditionally used by locals during winter in their everyday diet for their ability to tame fearful characters; raise energy; bring lovers together; boost sexual vitality and fertility; help with depression, anxiety and stress; and facilitate a good night's sleep during long winter nights.

The little seeds are used as a substitute for rennet in making cheese from the milk of domesticated yaks and goats, which thrive in the harsh climate of the Tibetan mountains.

Ballabh uprooted an ashwagandha shrub by easily pulling it from the ground. It had two finger-thick light-brown roots or 'legs', surrounded by many thin roots. He explained that this is one of the most popular herbs in Ayurvedic medicine, which allows his village to prosper.

With a wicked smile, Ballabh asked me to smell the root. It was unusual – pungent and unappetising. He explained that its name 'ashwa' (stallion) and 'gandha' (smell) suggests that it smells like a horse, and it is believed to transfer its sexual strength to its user, especially in the king's momos recipe, which he volunteered to cook for us on our return.

According to local legend, momos (a type of dumpling) were created by the first king of the Yarlung Dynasty, Nyatri Tsenpo, who descended from the sky in 127 BCE in order to recharge his power, as he planned to father as many children as he could before returning to the sky via a 'sky rope'. While the correct combination and purity of the ingredients is important, along with the particular ways of cooking techniques used, every Nepalese family has its own version of the recipe, which is usually prepared through the combined efforts of all family members.

Ballabh pinched off a finger-long tubular leaf from the almost leafless shrub nearby. While putting it into his mouth he explained that it was somlata (Ephedra) – one of the most sacred local plants.

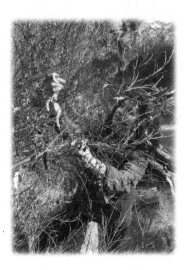

According to the local folktale, it was related to the Moon God and therefore used in the making of soma – a potent sex-stimulating drink, far better than any alcohol. Nomadic Nepalese tribes, who since ancient times had set temporary camps in remote parts of the forests, practice polyandry, where one woman marries several husbands. These women are usually very skilful in herbal medicine and are known to use somlata and ashwagandha to keep their men happy and satisfied.

Locals also enjoy the mild hallucinogenic effects of dried somlata in their teas and smoking mixes, however Ballabh preferred chewing freshly picked somlata leaves. Copying Ballabh, I put a small leaf into my mouth and chewed this bitter Nepalese marvel for an hour or so, before noticing a remarkable boost in my strength, a heightened sense of happiness and pleasant soul-soothing surges.

Here and there, I noticed the bright yellow flowers of the Mexican prickly poppy, which I remembered from our earlier travels to the Americas. Ballabh said that these poppies were good weeds, and the

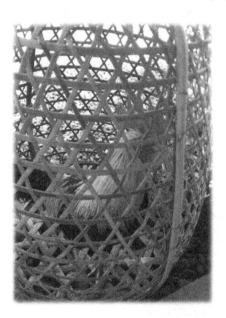

sap and dried flowers were used in ahrodisiac smoking mixes throughout India and Nepal.

Back at home, everyone was excited with the prospect of cooking momos. Ceremoniously, Ballabh allocated duties to every member of his family. Three of his younger children picked herbs and vegetables from their vegie patch. Their older brother caught a large red rooster, destined to be an ingredient in the ancient aphrodisiac recipe, which his wife then plucked and cleaned. The brightly dressed twelve-year-old daughter fetched some fresh water from the nearby river, which she then carried back home in a large jug, set in a cane basket attached by a ribbon to her head.

I was given the task of milling whole wheat into flour, using an old-fashioned stone grinder. The flour was soon skilfully turned into elastic dough by Ballabh's wife. Then, with a special momos-pinching technique, each dumpling was elaborately folded a certain way with no less than thirty-three pleats. Everyone, including my husband, was happy to give it a try, and we ended up with batch of 150 or so cute momos.

The ready-to-be-cooked momos were placed on oiled trays in the multi-deck steamer, which was set on top of a pot of boiling water. The pot rested comfortably on a metal tripod above the fire, which was set up in a square pit in the middle of the house.

Delicious aromas tortured our stomachs for thirty more minutes, and our excitement and appetites built to the extreme. Finally, we all sat down on comfortable, colourful wool-filled cushions around a low table to enjoy the juicy momos served in an aromatic broth – heavy and potent for the adults and clear chicken soup for the kids.

After the meal, we drank tea and ate candied ashwagandha fruit, and smoked a mix of tobacco and another local hallucinogenic stimulant – wild Mexican prickly poppy (Argemone mexicana), which locals forage for in late spring on the Nepalese slopes of the majestic Everest Mountain – the natural border between Nepal and China.

That night, my husband and I enjoyed the most delightful libido-awakening powers of the momos, and had highly erotic and euphoric dreams filled with lust and heightened sensuality, which stayed with us for several more days. Everything that Ballabh promised was delivered and more – a delightful experience!

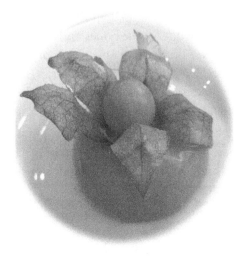

Ballabh's Momos

This complex dish is great for cooking parties, where friends can share the preparations and the excitement of the whole delightful experience.

> 5 cups wholemeal plain flour
> 2 cups cold water (add a little more if this is not enough)
> 4 onions, medium
> 50g ginger, fresh and chopped
> 100g ashwagandha berries, dried
> 100g ashwagandha root, dried or powdered
> 6 cloves of garlic
> 2 tablespoons of guduchi, dried leaves
> 1 bunch of cilantro (coriander)
> 1 chili, fresh
> soy sauce
> 1 chicken, fresh (preferably a rooster, as they are considered to be a symbol of sexuality, fertility and potency worldwide, with their cocks being the most potent part. Vegetarians can replace the chicken with a mix of chopped shiitake mushrooms and hard-set tofu.)

Serves 6

Make a hard dough using flour and water. Knead until smooth and flexible (if required, add some more water). Cover dough with a slightly wet, clean towel and let it rest for thirty minutes.

Debone the fresh chicken (save the bones and rooster's comb) and chop it into very small pieces. Add finely chopped 3 ½ onions, garlic, cilantro (save the roots), chopped dried ashwagandha berries, three tablespoons of soy sauce and three tablespoons of cold water, and dried guduchi leaves. Mix well using hands. Cover and let stand next to the dough.

Place washed chicken bones and comb into the pot. Cover with 1 litre of cold water and add remaining ½ chopped onion, cilantro roots, whole chili and ashwagandha roots. Cover with lid and slow boil until your momos are almost ready to be served.

Roll ¼ of the dough into a 2-inch thick sausage. Pinch off a small ball of dough and roll it in your palms until you have a smooth ball, then flatten it out into a circle, making the edges thinner than the middle.

Hold circle of dough in one hand and place a tablespoonful of filling in the centre with the other. Pinch the edge of the dough together above the centre just enough to make a small fold between your thumb and forefinger. Continue pinching around the circle little by little, keeping your thumb in place, and continuing along the edge of the circle with your forefinger, grabbing the next little piece of dough, and pinching the whole edge of the circle into one spot until you come back to where you started. Close the hole with a final pinch. Brush base of each momo with vegetable oil and place them on the steamer's trays – as many as will fit without touching each other. Steam for ten to twelve minutes.

Drain chicken bouillon through the sieve, cut rooster's comb into as many parts as there are males at the table, adjust taste with soy sauce and pour into the soup plates. Place eight to ten momos on each plate and decorate with the slice of rooster's comb (for men) and a streak of cilantro. Serve hot accompanied by soy sauce. Take care with the first bite as momos' hot juice can burn the tongue … then wait for the sensation of culinary orgasm to kick in and awaken your sexual desire.

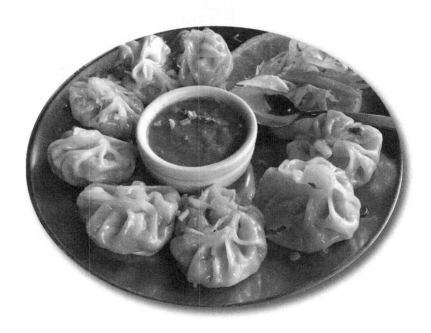

Legend: Never Fight Horny Man

When powerful Persia stretched from India to Ethiopia, there lived a very handsome king, Ahasuerus, also known as Xerxes. His first wife, the green-eyed Vashti, was well known for her stunning beauty – and her bad manipulative character. Unable to conceive a child, she hated all of Xerxes' other wives, and often secretly entertained herself by torturing them and drowning their children, or humiliating the slaves by forcing them to work naked with ash-smudged faces and genitals.

The slave Mordecai, who worked in the palace's kitchen as a cook, overheard Vashti plotting her latest murderous entertainment, this time against the Jews. He discussed it with his niece Esther, who supplied the king's kitchen with locally foraged herbs.

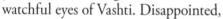

Together they came up with a plan, according to which the beautiful Esther would present the king with a large basket of valuable aphrodisiacs as a gift during his famous 180-day royal feast in Susa, and in return ask for protection. However, on the day of the feast she couldn't present it to the king under the watchful eyes of Vashti. Disappointed, Esther went to the kitchen and asked her uncle to use it in the king's favourite dish – lamb heads and testicles.

As per royal custom, during the feast, the king's friends, royal princes and all the top men of the kingdom were allowed to admire the splendour of the royal harem, where no expense was spared. The sexually over-excited king asked Vashti to dance before his guests, wearing just her jewelled royal crown.

The delighted men relaxed on the gold silk-cushioned couches in the courtyard, paved with white marble, rare red stones and blue turquoise, anticipating the sensual show. However Vashti refused the king's order.

Burning with desire to show off his wife's beauty, the king was humiliated, furious and embarrassed. He sought advice from his ministers, who quickly decided that – since the queen had publicly disobeyed her husband – all the wives of Persia might also revolt against their husbands.

The king ordered seven eunuchs to bring his disobedient wife before his eyes. Horny and unsatisfied, and most importantly insulted and humiliated in front of all the men of his kingdom, Ahasuerus took the crown off Vashti's head and banished her from his palace. Then, he looked around and noticing pretty Esther among his slaves, put it on Esther's head in front of all his guests, making her his queen. The rest is history …

Recipe:

1 lamb shoulder (deboned, approx 2kg) or 3 lamb heads and 6 testicles

100g ashwagandha powder

20g clove powder

1 parsnip, large

3 eggplants

1 garlic head

4 tablespoons of olive oil

1 tablespoon of sea salt

100g bread crust

1 nutmeg, grated

6 oregano sprigs, fresh (or 10g dried)

1 bunch of parsley

2 rosemary sprigs, fresh

½ bunch of basil, fresh

100g cream or butter

1 pomegranate

Mix ashwagandha roots, clove and nutmeg powder with 200ml of cold water. Rub lamb with this mixture, place on the roasting tray, cover and let stand in a cool place overnight.

Pre-heat oven to 170°C. Peel and chop parsnips and eggplants into large wedges. Blend salt, basil, bread crust, olive oil, onion and parsley into a green paste.

Cover marinated lamb all over with the paste, and sprinkle with rosemary leaves. Place lamb into preheated oven for two hours, baste every fifteen minutes. Place parsnip, eggplant and whole garlic head around the lamb, wrap the foil over the hot roasting dish and bake for forty-five more minutes.

Take lamb out of the oven; let stand for five minutes before unwrapping. Squeeze roasted garlic into a cup, add thick cream and cooking liquids from the baking tray, and salt and black pepper to taste. Whip together into a thick sauce, then strain through a fine sieve and serve with roast lamb, torn in pieces by hand, surrounded by parsnips, and decorated with parsley and pomegranate.

Eat with your hands; embrace the sensual feelings and delicious lust.

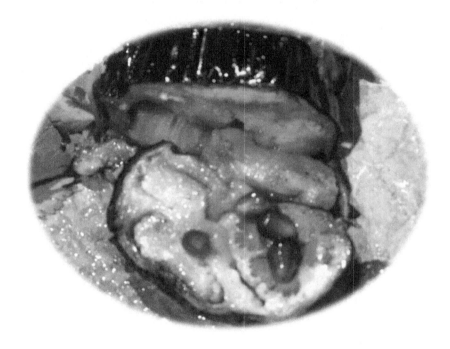

Maca - Peru

Lepidium meyenii (Latin) or Peruvian Ginseng

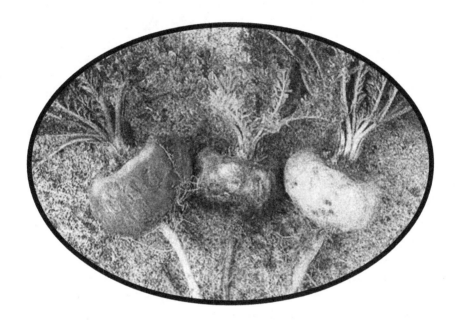

This tasty vegetable root contains large amount of biologically active elements, minerals and vitamins, which with regular use intensifies libido and stabilizes sexual conduct.

Dr. V.L.Zeltser

Sixteenth-century Spanish chronicles mention that Pre-Columbian Aztecs used maca and other aphrodisiacs, as well as a number of anaphrodisiacs, to modulate their sexuality or to gain the affection of a desired person.

While in Barcelona, we visited the famous Central Market, where I boldly asked one of the spice traders if he stocked any aphrodisiacs. With a meaningful smile, the enigmatic, unshaven Alejandro laid out three packets on the countertop and explained that they were aphrodisiacs which had been used in Spain for almost 500 years. He also said that they were made from the wild Peruvian vegetable, maca, originally introduced to Spain in the fifteenth century by the Spanish conquistadors of the Incan Empire.

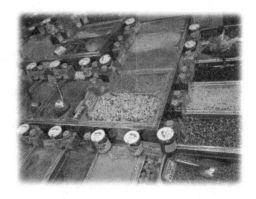

According to historical records, among the many things Spanish adventurers brought to the land of the Aztecs was European livestock, which did not reproduce well at the high altitudes of Peru. Friendly Incans suggested feeding their animals maca, which they used as a fertility aid for themselves and their animals.

Soon after, this resulted in a remarkable surplus of cattle, making the conquistadors realise maca's true value. They immediately imposed an annual maca tax on the local communities and exported it to Spain, from where it was distributed throughout Europe and Africa as a panacea and aphrodisiac worth its weight in gold.

My husband and I purchased all three of Alejandro's aphrodisiacs and rushed to our rented apartment anxious to try them. The recipes on the packs (tea, protein balls, smoothies, paste, pancakes and hot chocolate) were easy to make and quite tasty, however none of them produced any noticeable aphrodisiac effects.

Where did we go wrong? Could so many people be wrong for so long?! Or perhaps maca's magic worked only on cattle? To answer these questions we decided to go to Peru and personally test maca at its full strength, grown in its original habitat in the wild.

By a twist of fate, that night at a restaurant we spotted on the menu a dish made with Peruvian maca and the genitals of a bull killed at the corrida, but we didn't eat it on that occasion. A few years later, we dared to try it when we saw it again at a small restaurant in Bolivia, advertised as 'para machos el viagra criollos' (Spanish viagra for males).

Our English-speaking guide in Peru was Carlos Fernandez, a professional botanist. Armed with a small spade, he met us at the entrance to the Huayllay National Sanctuary in the Peruvian district of Pasco.

The land was covered with incredible natural rock formations, among which grew certain native plants. According to Carlos, cultivated maca is a staple food for Peruvians. However wild maca, known for its potency, can only be found at high altitudes, where it's not as accessible to foragers and wild animals.

Wild maca is highly regarded by the locals, as it is known to produce much stronger aphrodisiac effects due to the higher content of valuable sugars, protein, starches and essential nutrients, especially iodine and iron. High demand for the plant has resulted in widespread maca cultivation and high yields, which naturally comes at the cost of its potency.

As a child, Carlos remembered multiple stony maca fields around Cusco where it was grown for personal use, local markets and export. In order to preserve Peruvian rights on maca, and to prevent it being grown anywhere else in the world, the government forbade the export of maca other than in powdered form.

However, a few years ago, although protected by the international Nagoya Protocol, maca seeds were stolen by the 'Pirates del Oriente' (Asian entrepreneurs), who genetically modified the seeds for profiteering commercial purposes. This new lookalike maca vegetable does not contain any of wild maca's valuable medicinal properties, but it has flooded the market and caused a sharp decline in demand and resulting economic hardship for Peruvian farmers.

The aphrodisiac properties of wild maca are attributed to its ability to adapt to the hardships of the high altitudes – winds, cold winters, hot summers and stony soil – and its ability to store its magic powers in its plump roots, which later get passed on to its users.

Science has now reinforced what wild animals and the ancient Incans intuitively learned about this potent underground vegetable, and proved it's efficiency in triggering the body's own mechanisms to produce hormonal balance and increased sexual energy.

After hours of walking up a hill among beautiful flowering cactus clusters, my husband and I felt totally exhausted, while Carlos, who was in his eighties, was fresh and chirpy. Perhaps it was due to his love of maca?!

Finally, we climbed up to one of the highest plateaus, where wild maca was flourishing in abundance. Carlos carefully dug into the stony ground on one side of the maca plant to see if its root had reached the right size.

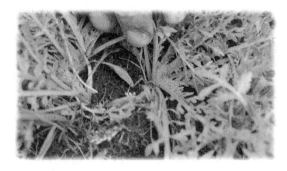

After a quick assessment, he pulled the pink root out and put it in the basket. My husband took over Carlos' spade and easily unearthed black, cream and hot-pink maca. In fact, it was even easier to pull them out of the ground by hand.

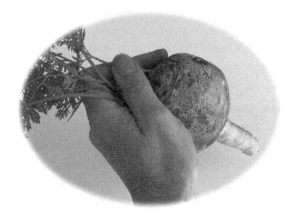

These colourful, plump, mustard-family roots looked like a hybrid of radish, parsnip and turnip, with similar thin skin and a bunch of green leaves on top.

On our return to Lima, Carlos introduced us to his friend Andres, who cooked our trophy tubers in his backyard overlooking the mountains, using his family's pachamanca recipe, which also included a reenactment of an ancient Incan sacred ritual for returning produce to the goddess of fertility – Pachamama (Mother Earth).

Andres' Pachamanca

While we enjoyed some *chicha de tora*, a delicious corn beer, Andres quickly built fire in the middle of his huatia (underground oven), which was simply a square ditch in the ground lined with rocks, with signs of having been used many times before. Then he placed an old iron grill on top and covered it with volcanic boulders.

While Andres was busy preparing the ingredients, we looked after heating the stones, which had to be occasionally slapped with a bunch of wet tree branches. The fumes of the burning wood, the leaves and the grass, mixed with the ancient rustic corn beer, produced a euphoric effect.

Carlos, also liberated by the chicha, warned us that the high level of amino acids in the pachamanca could escalate our sexual arousal beyond our expectations. Indigenous Incas used mashua – another Peruvian wonder plant known to suppress libido – to balance the maca's effects. Anecdotally, Peruvian wives purposely add mashua into their husbands' meals if they intend to travel alone.

When the fire had burned down, Andres pushed the hot stones to the side and removed the ashes from the ditch. In accordance with the ritual, he then ceremonially scattered thirteen fresh coco leaves (thirteen was the number of original Mayan gods) into the blazing hole, followed by local potatoes and whole onions, which he covered with hot stones.

The next layer consisted of large pieces of beef, pork and chicken marinated in red chilies, *huacatay* (Peruvian black mint), paprika, cumin, marjoram, thyme, turmeric, salt, corn beer and sliced tomatoes.

This next layer was also covered with blazing hot stones, on top of which our treasured wild maca was placed together with sliced pineapple, arracacha (a colourful carrot family plant) and ahipa (the root of the yam bean plant). A cute lidded sauce-pot, filled with a mixture of grated cheese and chopped local herbs, went into the corner to capture the heat of the escaping steam and melt into a delicious sauce.

Finally, everything was covered by a mass of fresh green herbs, with its aromatic sweat dripping down between the hot salted stones onto the food inside, making it moist and tasty. To capture every bit of the valuable steam, Andres sealed the oven with some old wet newspapers and cloths, secured on top with two buckets of dirt.

After about two hours, an amazing aroma emanated from the oven, signalling that the food was ready to be excavated! Remarkably all ingredients were perfectly cooked. Layer by layer, the colourful food was served on large platters, in a generous buffet-style dinner. The delicious tangy caramelised maca and the tender lamb with its butterscotch aroma dipped in the hot cheesy sauce made our jolly chicha-fuelled company feel revitalised, cheerful and sexually charged. We set there for hours exchanging jokes, then eating and drinking again.

Unfortunately I'm unable to provide exact quantities of ingredients for this recipe, as most of the ingredients were measured only by the handful.

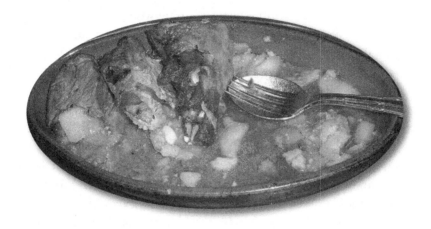

Legend: Fair Exchange

Five hundred years ago in the highlands of the Peruvian mountains, the Incan Empire prospered. It was as famous for its affluence as it was for its arm y of brutal warriors with their supernatural strength, resilience, stamina and enormous sexual appetite.

For centuries, many people tried to uncover their secret, but instead found their death, until King Atahualpa agreed to exchange the secret recipe with the Spanish conquistador Francisco Pizarro for twelve horses – animals yet unknown to the Incans.

The small Spanish army, weakened by extensive travelling, was re-charged by the Incan recipe, and within just a few months, had conquered the entire Incan Empire. After executing the thirteenth – and last – king of the Incans, they shipped all the Incan's gold to Spain and imposed hefty taxes on maca, which became popular in Europe as a miracle aphrodisiac from the New World.

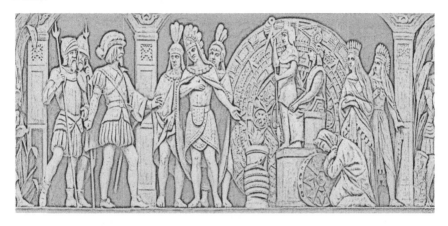

2 boiled maca root (or 4 tablespoons of dried maca powder)
250ml tomato juice
100g lucuma fruit pulp ('the last gold of the Incans', fresh mango can be used instead).
1 green or yellow capsicum
3 eggs
100g beef, turkey or chicken flesh, fully cooked
cayenne pepper (to taste)
sea salt (to taste)
100ml chicha de jora or vodka (optional)

<u>Garnish</u>
2 cucumbers, deseeded from the top and cut into thick rings
2 celery sticks, fresh
½ bunch of dill
12 ice cubes

Serves 4

Using blender, turn all ingredients (except cucumbers, dill and celery) into a smooth paste. Place this paste into the shaker and add chicha de jora, or vodka if you would like your drinks to be stronger. Shake vigorously for three minutes.

Pour into large glasses, add three ice cubes to each glass, and garnish with cucumber rings and dill sitting on the celery sticks. Eat by using celery stick instead of spoon.

This refreshment is an effective energy boost, especially on sultry summer evenings during lovemaking intermissions.

Damiana - USA

Turnera aphrodisiaca (Latin) or Mexican Holly

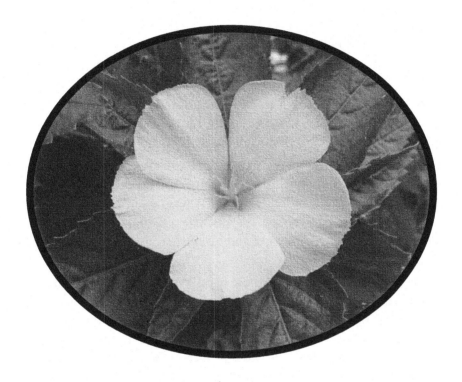

This plant contains number of alkaloids, that produce amatory effects through its direct impact on sex organs, nerves and blood circulation, as well as on psyche, producing a marijuana-like euphoria.

Dr. V.L.Zeltser

My fascination with the mysterious world of aphrodisiacs has not only opened an unexpected side of life for me, taught me about history and given me the opportunity to have some truly amazing experiences, it has also led me to meet many interesting people, who have shared their aphrodisiac experiences and knowledge. This story is about one of these encounters, which happened in the US, while my husband and I were on our saw palmetto expedition at the Canaveral Coast reserve.

We flew to Houston, Texas, intending to drive along the Gulf of Mexico to Jacksonville. We were due to meet there with a local forager, who had volunteered to be our guide to the Canaveral National Seashore in Florida, where we planned to collect some wild saw palmetto palm fruit.

On our way we stopped at many beautiful country towns, where people still appreciate and respect nature, but we lost our way and ended up in the small coastal town of Galveston late in the evening.

Tired and hungry, we were happy to spot a small seafood restaurant nearby which was still open. After ordering some delicious local seafood, we retired with a bottle of local beer. There was no one else at the restaurant and while he cooked, the talkative restaurant owner Martin told us about his town, its people and his life here as a second generation Mexican.

When he heard about the purpose of our trip, he became excited as he recalled chewing saw palmetto fruit with his schoolmates. Then, with a mysterious smile, he took a plump bottle from the bar and poured its yellowish liquid in three shot-glasses, commenting that this was his own aphrodisiac love liqueur, made from the local shrub, damiana. He swore it never failed to make him, his wife and their friends feel relaxed and horny. The recipe had always been in his family, who mainly used it as an antidepressant after they migrated to Texas from Mexico some fifty years ago.

We drank a few shots of Martin's bitter liqueur, but to our disappointment, felt only the effects of the alcohol. While we ate our seafood, the chatty Martin could not stop sharing his fascination with damiana.

According to him, since pre-historic times, this plant has been highly regarded for its effectiveness and was consecrated to the ancient love goddess Erzulie during spiritual and voodoo rituals.

Mexican psychics inhale smoke from incense made from damiana leaves and flowers mixed with bay leaves and sandalwood to heighten their visions, while shamans use it in their love magic. Martin told us many of his friends smoked handmade damiana joints (a mixture of dried leaves and tobacco) as a recreational substitute for marijuana, which induced a pleasant state of euphoria and meditation, provoked lust, and fought premature ejaculation, impotence and frigidity. In the old days, damiana was commonly added to cattle feed to stimulate fertility.

Ancient Aztec women used damiana in different combinations in their cooking to stimulate lovemaking in their men, to induce abortion and to prevent bedwetting in children. Even today, damiana is still widely used by indigenous people of North America to enhance sex and fertility.

For dessert, Martin gave us a long drink of iced tea made with honey and, you guessed it, damiana, which was a big mistake, as after approximately two hours we sank into a pleasant yet dynamic euphoria, as if we had ingested marijuana and coca. We ended up walking on the beach kissing and hugging till sunrise, unable to sleep all night.

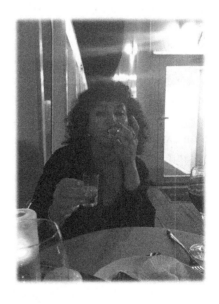

Our research also indicated that damiana – native to Mexico – is an important part of Mexican culture and has been protected by a ban on the exportation of live plants.

Next morning, we went back to see the friendly Martin, who agreed to not only share his aphrodisiac secret recipe with us, but to take us to the place where he usually collected damiana for his love liqueur.

We drove for over two hours in his huge, robust Grand Cherokee Jeep towards Corpus Christi, located close to the Mexican border, where damiana bushes were supposed to grow on the side of the road like weeds.

The best time to pick damiana leaves and flowers is in mid to late summer. While fresh damiana is more effective, it also works well after being dried in the shade, as direct heat destroys the valuable alkaloids responsible for increasing blood flow to the genitals, which stimulates libido and produces feelings of euphoria.

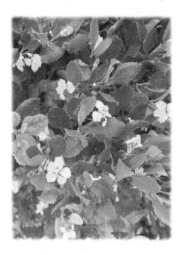

Soon we stopped on a curve of the road where we spotted many damiana shrubs with their small yellow flowers. There in the dry, hot climate of Texas in the rocky Rio Grande Valley bloomed the evergreen damiana bush, looking definitely at home. I crushed a few shiny leaves in my palm and they gave off a pleasant, aromatic woody scent, which obviously was there due to the presence of the essential oil.

Martin prompted us to collect leaves and head back to the vehicle as quickly as possible, as if we were stealing them, which irritated us. But we soon understood only too well when a military vehicle arrived with two armed border patrol officers! They were very suspicious about this trio collecting leaves from the bushes next to the Mexican border, and grilled us for fifteen minutes under the hot Texan sun before checking our passports and letting us go. It wasn't pleasant, but we still had our trophy in Martin's trunk.

After deliciously potent pink grapefruit and shellfish salad at Martin's joint, we went to the back of his restaurant to watch the ancient love liqueur being prepared.

There we met Martin's wife Paula, who offered us her damiana recipe for a potent 'feel good' tea for women, which she said induced erotic euphoria and helped to combat the symptoms of premenstrual tension or menopause.

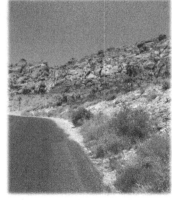

Martin's Love Liqueur

60g damiana leaves, fresh (or 25g dry)

3cm galangal root (or young ginger)

1 teaspoon of nutmeg powder

750ml vodka or white rum

100g agave syrup (or cold-pressed honey)

1 vanilla bean (or ½ lemon, zested)

100ml mineral or filtered water

Serves 20

Wash and finely chop damiana leaves. Place in large jar, add nutmeg powder and sliced galangal root, and cover with alcohol. Tighten lid and let stand in direct sun for two days.

Strain liquid into another jar and place in a cool spot. Cover the residue with water and let it steep overnight. Then strain liquid through a fine sieve lined with cheesecloth, and mix with agave syrup. Combine liquid with alcoholic extract.

Cut vanilla bean lengthwise and insert into a clean glass bottle (approximately one litre volume), top it up with love liqueur, cap and store in a cool, dark place.

Please be aware that this drink is potent for both sexes. Share with someone special. Serve as libido shots or mixed with champagne as a romantic pick-me-up drink.

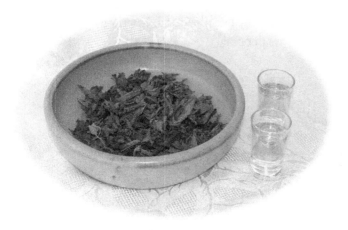

Paula's 'Feel Good' Tea

30g damiana leaves, dried and rubbed
50g wild yam powder
1 litre water, boiling hot

Mix damiana and wild yam powder into one litre of hot water. Let brew for fifteen minutes. Strain, add some honey or brown sugar, fresh mint and lemon to taste. Serve warm or cold with ice.

Martin's Potent Grapefruit and Shellfish Salad

2 pink grapefruits
1 lettuce, shredded
1 cucumber, deseeded and diced
200g prawns, cooked and peeled
300g crab meat, cooked
5 tablespoons of sour cream
1 tablespoons of Dijon wholegrain mustard
½ lime, juiced
2 tablespoons of Martin's love liqueur
Salt and cayenne pepper to taste

Serves 4

Cut grapefruit in half and scoop out the segments creating serving bowls. Remove seeds and reserve the juice. Chop the segments, flake crab meat and combine with half of the shredded lettuce, prawn and cucumber. Mix sour cream, mustard, Martin's love liqueur, lime and reserved grapefruit juice. Evenly distribute left-over lettuce in the grapefruit shells and top up with seafood. Spoon over the dressing and sprinkle with cayenne pepper.

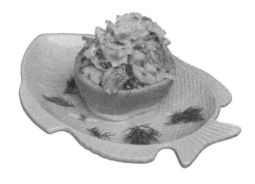

Legend: Cookies for the King

'I have found it impossible to carry the heavy burden of responsibility and to discharge my duties as king as I would wish to do without the help and support of the woman I love,' said King Edward VIII in his abdication speech in 1936.

No one could ever explain why, just six months before his coronation as king of the United Kingdom and the Dominions of the British Commonwealth and as emperor of India, the heir to the British crown chose love – for the allegedly unsuitable, twice-divorced American woman, Wallis Simpson – over the throne of England with its power, riches and royal obligations.

This scandalous love story puzzled many people for almost a century. Was it simply the love of two lonely souls from completely different backgrounds, or was it witchcraft, hypnosis or something even more sinister?

Love did not sound convincing enough, and at the time, there were rumours about the American woman bewitching the king. The gossip was allegedly started by one of Wallis' two ex-husbands, who stated that in the past she had been known to use love drugs – in particular, the Mayan plant damiana.

She believed that this ancient botanical gave her power over men's minds, by rousing unmanageable passion and lust in them for her, and she was known to use it in cocktails, smoking blends – where tobacco was mixed with orange blossoms or other aromatic grass – cooking and her famous Royal Cookies, allegedly created for her royal sweetheart.

Recipe:

30g damiana leaves, dried
1 egg
6 tablespoons raw honey or brown sugar
50g walnuts, chopped (or pine nuts)
50g raisins (or sultanas)
120g unsalted butter (or coconut cream)
pinch sea salt
60ml water
1 vanilla bean (or 10ml of vanilla extract)
200g plain white flour
50g icing sugar (optional)

Pre-heat oven to 190°C. Pound dry damiana leaves into dust, sieve over the mixing bowl, add an egg, pinch of salt, honey, vanilla bean seeds and water, and mix well. Cover mixture and let it stand for ten minutes in a cool place.

Mix in unsalted softened butter, then flour. When the mixture looks homogeneous, add walnuts and sultanas and knead mixture into soft dough.

Form twenty thick cookies of any shape and size you desire, place them on the baking tray lined with baking paper, and pop into oven for ten to twelve minutes or until golden-brown.

When at room temperature, dust cookies with icing sugar and hide in the cookie jar with an air-tight lid. Enjoy as an afternoon treat with glass of champagne, coffee or tea.

One or two cookies per person should be enough to produce a pleasantly stimulating sensual high that will kick in after an hour or so and will will last few hours thereafter.

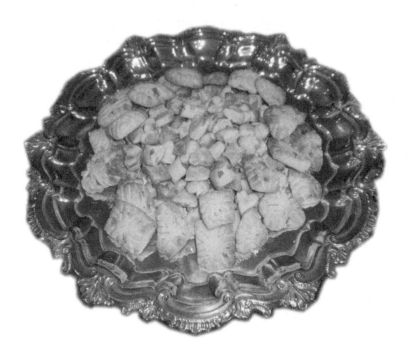

Tongkat Ali – Indonesia

Eurycoma longifolia (Latin), also known as Long Jack

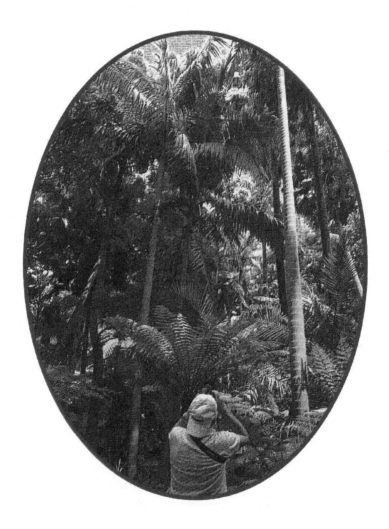

High levels of chemical compound glyco saponins and eurypeptides brand Tongkat Ali plant as perfect natural remedy for support of male hormonal balance (including testosterone levels), sex drive and performance.

Dr. V.L.Zeltser

A few years ago at our local pharmacy, I noticed an advertisement for some miraculous capsules made of tongkat ali root. It promised the miraculous regeneration of 'sexy muscles', the speedy production of testosterone, and resilience to stress. The helpful shop assistant explained that this product had neem made in Indonesia from the roots of a tree, native to its rainforests.

These claims were supported by scientific studies and ancient pharmacopoeia books, which also said the indigenous people of Southeast Asian countries had used it for centuries. My extensive research backed up most of these facts and claims, and fuelled my desire to find tongkat ali in the wild, where I could experience its powers at full strength.

Our hotel in Bali was made entirely from bamboo and set in close proximity to the luscious rainforest and rice terraces on the evergreen hills. Our concierge, Pastor, was surprised to hear about my interest in the tongkat ali tree.

He told me that his parents and grandparents used the roots of 'long jack' (the local name) to make brew, which was used almost every day as a cold or hot drink and in cooking. The bitter amber brew was made to an ancient recipe from the real roots of the tree, as the locals believed that capsules, sold at the pharmacies, were not as effective.

However, it seemed the younger generation preferred to buy processed tongkat ali root from pharmacies, roadside hawkers or supermarkets, where it was sold in tea bags. Pastor also said some restaurants offer tongkat ali root powder mixed with coffee or other beverages. He warned me about the many fake products sold to naïve tourists and suggested we look for real thing at the Chinese herbal shop at the local day-market.

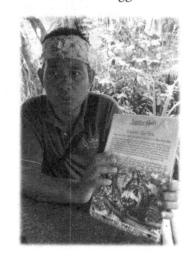

Unfortunately the Chinese herbal shop at this tourist-hungry market only had powdered roots in stock. The coffee shop next door was selling tongkat ali coffee, which I thought must have been fake as it did not produce any effects on my husband or me.

We also came across another exotic coffee called Kopi Luwak. It was claimed that this coffee had been made out of partially digested coffee beans, defecated by Asian palm civets, and it was advertised as a sexual stimulant. I was aware that both African and Asian civet cats were famed for their sex glands, which produce one of the strongest pheromones known, so I decided to taste test this expensive exotic coffee. To my disappointment, it was sour with an unpleasant smell, which was probably due to the fermentation process of the coffee beans in the civet's intestines. But, most importantly, it did not have any other effect on me than normal coffee would.

Dissatisfied, I complained to Pastor, who by that time managed to convince his friend Putra, a local forester, to take me and my husband foraging for tongkat ali in the local rainforest.

Next morning, the four of us drove into the massive green mountains. We passed many colourful small villages full of Hindu temples set among picturesque rice fields, dense jungles, huge Banyan trees and coconut palms.

Each village specialised in specific agriculture crops, art or music. The aroma of exotic tamarind, snake fruit, fragrant clove trees and bright-red flame trees, acacias and mangroves excited our senses. Cut flowers and tropical fruit decorated the many temples and shrines as offerings to the spirits of the ancestors and the Balinese gods – Brahma, Vishnu and Shiva.

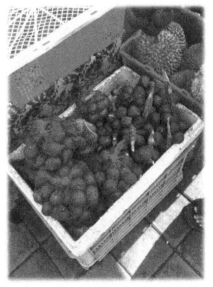

Along the way, the easygoing Putra told us about Balinese culture and the importance of tongkat ali (known now as 'Asian viagra') to the indigenous Balinese, who for centuries used it to stimulate blood surges to men's genitals, as a cure for malaria, for fertility, and to strengthen overall health.

When Putra got tired of talking, Pastor took over, telling us intimate facts about Balinese culture, Buddhism, local traditions and life in the villages, which cast a different perspective on this stunning island. He explained that the lucky Putra, who worked as a forester for the local municipality, had also inherited his father's land and grew vegetables

119

which family members sold at the local market to support their large household.

On both sides of the road, local vendors, armed with a few words from many different languages, sold local fruit, petrol in plastic bottles and homemade Arak, a cloudy, highly alcoholic drink which was popular among young tourists. It was invented by Indonesian Buddhists, who made it from fermented glutinous rice or sugar palm sap, for use in ritual ceremonies.

Finally, we stopped and ventured on foot further into the humid, bird-filled jungle. We passed by volcanic cones tightly covered with luscious green vines, flowering lianas, wild jasmine, colourful hibiscus and bougainvillea. The warm air was heavy with the intoxicating floral scent of magnolia mixed with frangipani, orchids and grass.

Putra led our expedition confidently through the jungle to the spot where he had harvested 'pasak bumi' (tongkat ali in Indonesian) before. There were many similar trees growing, however – according to Putra – only one species out of the five that belonged to this family was an aphrodisiac. Finally, he spotted what he was looking for.

It was a tall, thin tree, probably three to four years old, with a slim, straight trunk decorated with a canopy of green oblong leaves on short branches, which formed an umbrella at the top.

Apparently it was a male tree, which means the roots were more valuable than the female tree, as it was far more potent. Using a small shovel, Putra quickly dug around the tree, baring the top part of the roots. Then he tied a rope around it and linked it back to the trunk, creating a loop.

Using a wooden stick for leverage, within five to ten minutes Putra pulled the tree out of the moist sandy ground, managing not to damage any of its valuable, light-brown forked roots.

While we walked back to the car, I felt sorry for the rest of the tree, which had been left behind as waste, and yet no doubt it contained the same properties as its roots, just in a smaller concentration. Pastor assured me that native animals like monkeys, civets, mousedeer, barking deer and the jungle itself would make good use of it, and that one should always share everything with nature.

Putra boasted that he had never been sick in his life, as he regularly drank tongkat ali tea, which his grandfather introduced him to when he was twelve months old, and he volunteered to prepare it for us on our return. Every family in Bali has its own secret recipe, supported by the legends, and their own private stories – such as the one about Putra's grandmother, who at sixty-two gave birth to his uncle, while her husband was well into his nineties!

Tired, intrigued and curious, we drove to Putra's village. His house was built in traditional Balinese style, with its front yard dedicated to the memory of his ancestors. After paying our respects, we stepped into the back garden full of bright-red flame-tree blossoms. The same flowers were delicately woven into the hair of Putra's three daughters.

After washing the roots under running water, Putra chopped them into two- to three-centimetre pieces, and dropped them into a pot of boiling water, which he simmered uncovered for approximately twenty minutes.

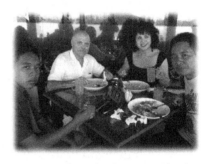

This produced a clear, yellowish bitter tea with a tarty taste that was pleasing to the palate, which was then strained and served in small tea cups. We experienced a pleasant thirty-minute herbal high, and a conscious dream-like state of happiness, explaining its centuries-old use in rituals.

The rest of the tea was used later in Putra's grandmother's stew, which also featured a retired red-feathered fighting rooster as an ingredient.

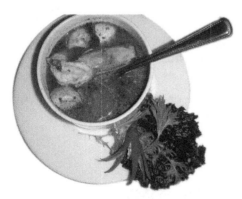

This rich, colourful dish had a strong piquant aroma and was served in large soup bowls with rice noodles and soft-shell crabs, decorated with sliced chili and cilantro.

And ... yes – it worked! Despite the increased air humidity our bodies, tired from the expedition, soon felt re-charged and ready for action, as if an energy producing burner had been installed inside. Our minds were clear and we felt sexually excited and happy to release some of this energy by copying Putra's daughters' sensual Balinese dance movements.

That night in the Balinese tropics was one of the most memorable sensual nights of our lives – with our wildest romantic dreams realised!

Putra's Stew

½ cup vegetable oil
1 chicken (rooster), organic or 500g of tempeh (vegan option)
1 onion, chopped
1 galangal, chopped
3 nettle roots, chopped
2 jimsonweed flowers
2 star anise pods
6 cardamom pods
20g cumin seeds, powdered
2 celery sticks, chopped
6 potatoes, peeled, cut in quarters
3 carrots, peeled and sliced
100g tongkat ali root, powder
500g morning glory shoots or flat rice noodles
4 chili, fresh (subject to personal preference)
1 bunch of cilantro
4 frangipani flowers (decoration)
4 tablespoons ketjap manis (sweet soy sauce)
1 teaspoon coconut blossom sugar

Serves 6

Place all ingredients in a deep clay pot, except chili, cilantro, frangipani blossoms and morning glory shoots. Cover with lid and pop into the oven for two hours at 170°C.

Serve over morning glory shoots with rice or noodles as a soup or stew, and decorate with sliced chili, cilantro and frangipani blossoms. The piquant bitterness of tongkat ali is pleasant and adds exotic undertones to this dish.

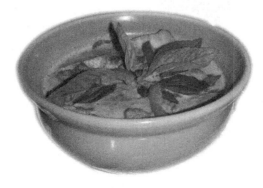

Legend: The Greatest Secret of Siam

Once upon a time in Siam, there lived a powerful ruler – King Rama II – who had seventy-two children and thirty-eight wives. When he died, his older son Jetta was crowned as Rama III. According to the Siamese tradition, he had to marry his father's wives and outnumber his father by having even more wives and children. It wasn't easy, and he died before fulfilling his royal obligations.

Then his younger brother, who was serving as a monk, stepped into his shoes, and was crowned as Phrachomklao Rama IV or Mongkut (monk-king). He quickly fathered eighty-two children with his thirty-nine official wives and almost nine-thousand concubines from all over the world, including those who had belonged to his father and brother.

The secret of his success was attributed to a secret tea, which he drank every day before going to bed. While serving as a monk, he had had to avoid some plants in order to keep his celibacy. Confronted by the challenge, he used his knowledge in reverse and came up with an effective potion, which enhanced his physique and sexuality – and allegedly enlarged his member. He kept this recipe in secret, and prepared it only behind closed doors, however his servants' curiosity and greed helped the world to learn about this effective invigorating recipe.

Recipe:

3 tablespoons of coriander seeds, pounded
100g tongkat ali root (shavings or powder)
¼ lime, zested
750ml brem (rice wine made from ketan sticky rice) or vodka
2g cinnamon powder
6 cloves
1 teaspoon of green Ceylon tea, heaped
100g honey (or brown sugar)
300ml water

Serves: 25

Lightly roast the tongkat ali root shavings or powder together with cinnamon, cloves and coriander. Grind all into a powder, then place into a jar and cover with brem. Add lime zest and cap tightly. Allow to steep for two weeks. Shake daily.

123

Strain mixture through cheesecloth into a clean glass jar. Keep the residue. Lightly warm up water in a small pot, adding the Ceylon tea and residue. Simmer for ten minutes, then strain, and mix in honey or brown sugar. When at room temperature, combine with alcoholic brew and cap tightly. Allow to age for two weeks.

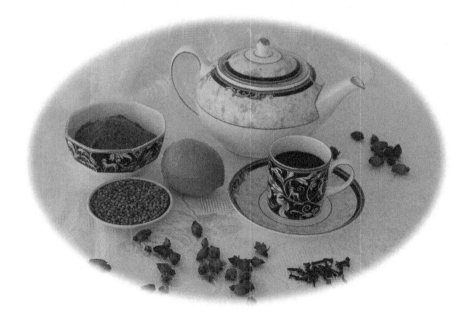

Mandrake – Italy

Mandragora officinarum (Latin) or Mandragora,
Love Apple, Crazy Apple

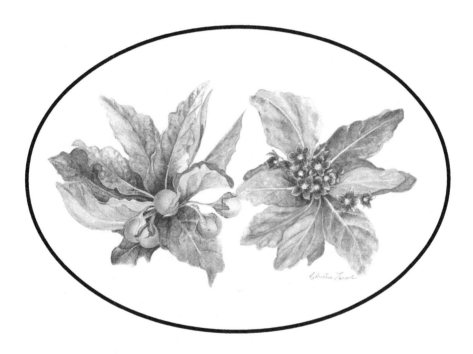

*The main active ingredients of this powerful narcotic and hypnotic plant
are tropanes – nervous system stimulants, which include, among others,
atropine and cocaine, that can produce hallucinations known as astral
travel experience.*   *Dr. V.L.Zeltser*

From ancient Middle Eastern medicinal books to African and European historical records and mythology, mandrake has been positioned as a mysterious aphrodisiac, able to deliver love, power, desire and even death. One of the oldest known aphrodisiacs, mandrake has been used for millennia in witchcraft, religious rituals and pharmacopoeia. People believed that its beneficial magical qualities included the escalation of sexual pleasure and emotional attachment.

The hairy root has been heralded in numerous books from the Bible to the poetry of King Solomon, and even in the works of Shakespeare. It was also used as a potent enchanted amulet, which attracted prosperity and success to its owners and protected them from the evil eye. Alexander the Great attributed his triumph to mandrake root, which he always carried with him.

Ancient civilisations in European and Eastern Asian countries used this mysterious root in medicine, love potions and rituals, or as a magic talisman to promote fertility, attract a lover or combat madness. It was also used to cure insomnia and various illnesses associated with the human mind. Its aromatic, fleshy orange fruits – not pleasant to my taste – were used as purgatives and anaesthetics. They were also fed to animals to induce a sleepy state before they were slaughtered.

The roots – which contain a high concentration of psychoactive alkaloids – were usually extracted and given to patients by Roman doctors to reduce pain and relax muscles before brutal surgeries or dental procedures. Even the dried leaves of mandrake, which contain very mild doses of hallucinogen, were used, as a bedroom incense or pot pourri to enhance psychoactive sexual experiences and excite desire.

While it is not known how this potent root loaded with narcotic compounds was discovered, I am inclined to think that its mysterious shape, resembling the human body, most definitely contributed to the initial interest in it. This of course was reinforced by the visible magic produced by one of the mandragora's chemicals – atropine, known to increase the heart rate and dilate the pupils of the eye, which was used by women to make their eyes look more attractive. Its value in the ancient world was so high that it was often faked by traders, who shaped different roots to look like mandrake, which – it is said anecdotally – worked as a placebo.

Despite centuries-old ghost stories and legends, deadly warnings and bizarre claims about mandrake's link to evil powers – for example, its seeds being the semen and blood of violently killed men – anxious people willingly resorted to its magic. Even now desperate lovers resort to this shaggy mystical root in the hope of materialising their dreams.

Intrigued and sceptical about mandrake's powers and the accuracy of the historical references, I decided to personally test mandrake's legendary aphrodisiac powers. It took me a while to find a spot in Europe where it can still be found growing in the wild – in Sicily.

The beautiful Vendicari coastal reserve, past Syracuse city, greeted us with unusually windy and rainy weather for May. We stayed at a cosy old hotel, located close to the ancient town of Lido di Noto. Angela Morrone, a bubbly local forager and school teacher, headed our mandrake expedition, explaining that according to the local tradition mandrake can only be harvested on a Friday following a full moon. Thus, we had three days to explore and admire the beautiful island of Sicily before the right harvesting time would come.

Angela picked us up at six am and, while driving us to the place where mandrakes grow in the wild, she told us about some amazing

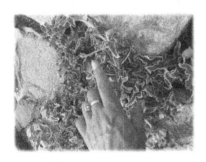

local legends, strange superstitions, mysteries and scary rituals, and she even promised to introduce us to the local witch.

We stopped at the picturesque rocky Vendicari seaside, and after a cup of strong sweet coffee from Angela's thermos, we followed her by foot.

Soon, I spotted a mandrake plant with three bright, glossy, gold-orange miniature fruit resting on the dried and welted large leaves. I picked up the tomato-like fruit and split it open. It contained many shiny yellow and light-brown seeds. I was overwhelmed by the pretty sight, and imagined how pretty this plant was in the early spring, when its bright purple blossoms clustered in the centre of its luscious green leaves. Angela suggested this plant was not worth pulling up, as it most probably only had a little root, and that we needed to look for plants with no less than six fruit.

As we walked deeper into the colourful wilderness, Angela regaled us with stories about this enigmatic ingredient of southern Italian witchcraft. Its popularity as an aphrodisiac in Catholic Sicily is owed to the Book of Genesis, where the love-hungry Rachel asks Leah to give her mandrake root, which her son Reuben found in the field.

Soon after, at the edge of the village, we spotted a large mandrake plant with nine golden apples, which according to Angela was large enough for the local witch to use in her famous magic confarreatio cake, also known as torta nuziale (bride's cake).

Silently, she took earplugs from her bag and pushed them into her ears, then made three circles around the plant and started digging it out, while telling us that – according to local beliefs – if mandrake is pulled from the earth, it shrieks, causing madness and death. While she did not believe in it herself, she still had to keep up appearances. To avoid this curse, locals had invented a special technique to safely harvest mandrake with the help of a black dog, which was tied to the plant and then – when called by its owner from a safe distance – would pull the plant out of the ground. It seems that the curse didn't work on dogs.

After few minutes, Angela unearthed about ten centimetres of the thick, skin-coloured root, but it was still firmly rooted in the stony ground. She kept on digging, however ten centimetres later, Angela accidently missed the ground and hurt her toe with a spade. The root was still far from being excavated and my husband came to the rescue.

He patiently dug into thick mud, which was oozing under his runners, until Angela said that it was time to pull the root out. With his back against the wind and his feet firmly placed on either side of the plant, he gripped the top of the root with both hands and yanked it with all his might to re-create the legendary shriek ... we heard a loud snap, followed by my own piercing shriek as I watched my husband fall over backwards in the mud, clutching the upper half of the mandrake root in his hands.

The root was shaped like a one-and-a-half legged man, and smelled of mud. It was not what we hoped for, but it was enough for the mandragora cake recipe, and we survived to tell the tale.

On our way to our meeting with the local buona strega (good witch), Angela warned us that witches could be vindictive if not treated with the highest respect. Captivated, curious and a little scared, we drove into the overgrown front yard of a large old house.

Angela walked inside Strega's house, while we were left in the car. Shortly, she came out and invited us in. To our disappointment, she was not an ugly old woman dressed in black rags, but a pleasant, forty-something Italian lady, who did not speak any English. The witch was holding our mandragora root away from her body and patting it, as if it were alive.

Angela explained that unfortunately confarreatio cake could not be made that day, as it required more ingredients than we had brought, however, in exchange for our root, Strega would be happy to let us try her mandrake love potion and tell us how the cake was made – but, of course, without revealing the secret ingredients.

Strega offered us some mandragora potion, which she poured into small glasses. It had a pleasant taste, somewhat like claret wine and dried fruit. Soon after, its magic powers kicked in and our vision became slightly distorted, our pupils enlarged and mouths dry, and we felt happy, relaxed, elated and sexually aroused. This phenomenon was attributed by my husband to the presence of atropine in the plant.

Happy with the result, Strega told us that since medieval times confarreatio cake had been used to bewitch desired lovers or to bind newlyweds for life. The ancient magic seemed to work, as in those days there was rather less divorce in Italy. Confarreatio cake is still regularly made for local women, who use it on their sluggish husbands or to attract a lover. It is baked only in the presence of the woman, who wishes to bind her man to her heart.

The ingredients include secret spices, black truffle, cocoa powder, borax, nuts and local dried fruits macerated in mandragora wine, grated mandrake root and other common ingredients like flour, eggs and honey, which are mixed in a certain order and proportion. Softly, Angela added that vaginal secretions were also used in the cake, which Strega forgot to mention.

The cake is baked in a small oven placed on a thick board over the loins of the totally naked woman wanting to attract the man. While she lies on the table, enduring five to seven kilograms of heavy load on her lower stomach, she is expected to repeat after Strega a magic spell, and tell her about her loved one.

When ready, the square-shaped cake is decorated with magic signs and it is the woman's responsibility to serve it to the right person. Frankly,

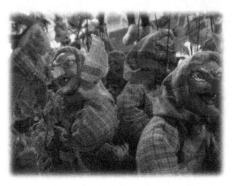

after hearing all that, I felt relieved at not being able to witness either the cake-making ritual or to eat it, and I have never attempted to re-create it at home, as I don't have enough knowledge of its chemistry and biology to get the handling and doses correct, so that I do not poison anyone with it.

Legend: Besos de Chocolate

The famous womaniser Don Juan devoted his entire life to conquering as many women's hearts as he could. Many of his stories found their way into literature and folklore, which often unjustly pictured him as an egoistic, shameless adulterer and cruel seducer, who broke many women's hearts – but no one ever mentioned how hard Don Juan had to work to get his rewards and how much his victims actually enjoyed his seduction. And most importantly, no one ever mentioned his own aphrodisiac invention – besos de chocolate (chocolate kisses).

In 1526 Don Juan received a letter from his friend, the Spanish conquistador Cortes. He informed Don Juan about his discovery of a potent aphrodisiac remedy in the New World, which the Aztec emperor Montezuma drank every night from golden goblets, which he called 'cacahuatl'. This magic bitter beverage made the old emperor euphoric and sexually excited, and also induced a state of desire, ecstasy and pleasure in his women. Cortes, knowing his friend's love inclinations, offered Don Juan the chance to be first to buy the beans from his merchant in Spain. Eager to try anything that worked on women in an amorous way, Don Juan paid a fortune for the cocoa beans.

The intuitive Don Juan turned Montezuma's bitter and peppery beverage into a delicious sweet treat, which pleased thousands of Spanish ladies, who fell in love with the chocolate and its inventor. It quickly became his trademark, and brought many blissful and memorable moments to his lovers, as well as helping them to justify their sins by blaming the chocolate for it! Dr Zeltser, my talented husband, was inspired by this story, which resulted yet in another deliciously potent aphrodisiac product - Cacao High capsules and electuaries.

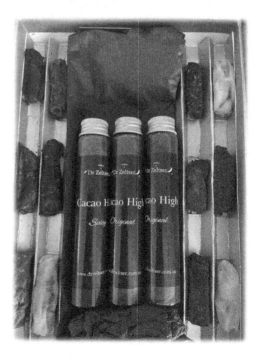

Don Juan's Chocolate Game

200g almonds (processed into 500ml of milk)
200g dark chocolate (or 130g honey, 10g vanilla extract and 70g cocoa powder)
40g corn flour
200ml port
pinch of chili powder
100g raspberries, blackberries or alpine strawberries
Pack of al mond biscotti

Place almond milk and chocolate (or all chocolate ingredients) into a small pot and bring it to simmer. Stir in corn flour dissolved in a little cold water until it totally dissolves and chocolate thickens to the consistency of sour cream. Take off the heat. Pour into a large, wide cup. Let it set for fifteen minutes. Mix berries into the chocolate cream, dust with some chili powder and serve with almond biscotti. Feed your lover with the almond biscotti dipped in chocolate, and try to fish out the berries using only the biscotti. Kiss every time it happens or come up with your own erotic games, like body painting.

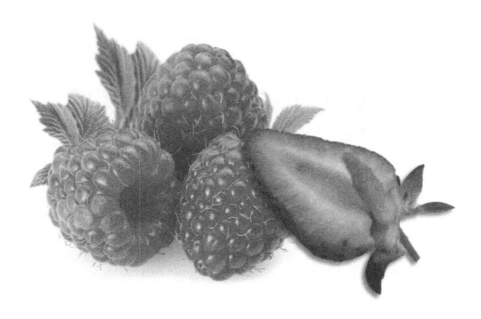

French Aphrodisiacs - France

The art of sensual cookery

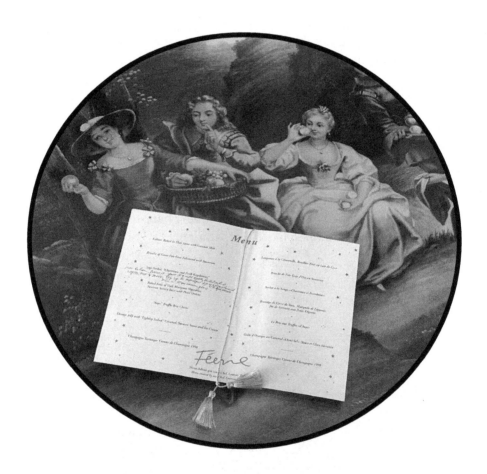

There is no real magic behind aphrodisiacs! It is simply a matter of mastering understanding and usage of the components that able to actively nourish and stimulate human senses. Aphrodisiacs shall not be restricted to enhancement of the physical act of love, but should cover a much broader spectrum of general well-being, behaviour and overall satisfaction with life.

Dr. V.L.Zeltser

While my taste buds prefer Mediterranean cuisine, my mind had always been fascinated by the complexity of French cuisine and its reputation for being romantic, erotic and libido stimulating. So many people cannot be wrong!

From the nineteenth century onwards, those who could afford to travel to France were inevitably hooked on the orgasmic and pleasure-awakening French cuisine. French cookery is known to tickle lovers' senses, which caused its fame around the world. It is well known that a good dinner at a French restaurant can put diners in a sensual romantic mood, and provoke and restore interest in Cupid's arrows.

Experienced French waiters entertain themselves by observing the magic changes that occur between diners before and after their meal … couples who were seemingly cold to each other at the start of an evening leave the restaurant with sizzling eyes, desperate for privacy.

Why? Is there a secret ingredient there? What do French chefs know and serve to make people feel that way? Trying to discover their secret, I combed through many French cookbooks including those of the most-celebrated French chefs – such as Marie-Antoine Carême, Auguste Escoffier and many more – however, I could not spot the secret ingredient or cooking technique that gave French cuisine its reputation as an

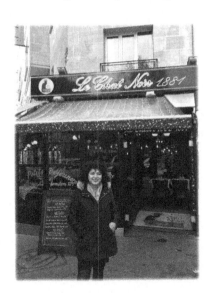

aphrodisiac – and one that seems to work for all people regardless of their race, religion or ethnic belonging! Thus, I went to France in search of the mysterious French aphrodisiac secrets.

It was late December, and the weather was crispy with the cold morning sun shining in a pale blue sky. I walked through the empty-at-that-hour Moulin Rouge, the legendary red-light district of Paris, famous for its cabarets, sex shops, private clubs, secluded secret doors and iconic restaurants.

I decided to stop at a small café for a short expresso, where I met a friendly shopkeeper, Gerome. He wasn't surprised to hear the reason for my trip to France, which only confirmed my suspicion about the existence of French aphrodisiacs.However, he reassured me that the secret behind French aphrodisiacs was simply the knowledge of how the human senses work and react to different foods, drinks, sounds and aromas.

From the fifteenth to the eighteenth centuries, the overindulged and prospering French court created great demand for things that could provide pleasure and stimulate the senses. It prompted many artists, perfumers, jewellers and chefs to innovate in all areas of art, cookery and fashion.

Talented chefs experimented with unusual ingredients, aromas and colours and then observed the emotional and bodily effects of their recipes on diners and adjusted their recipes to make them more effective. Armed with this knowledge they elevated simple cookery to the level of art, where food and drink was used as a tool to heighten sexual desire, seduce lovers, start wars or help to swing the minds of politicians.

During the French revolution, many indulgent aristocrats were beheaded, leaving countless orphaned chefs unemployed. In order to survive, many of them opened public eateries where they served their unique dishes and continued inventing even more effective recipes in order to withstand fierce competition. Hence, the secret of French cookery became available to the citizens of the French Republic and its curious tourists, who spread its fame around the world.

The culture of French restaurants became the standard for dining perfection in Europe and captured the attention of the world. Many chefs became rich and famous, and some of them were contracted by opulent houses, where they enjoyed royal treatment and high remuneration.

Diners, hungry for sensual experiences, travelled for months from many different countries just to experience the magic power of French cuisine at posh restaurants such as Maxims, La Tour d'Argent or Le Procope. This profitable phenomenon stimulated the creativity of French chefs even further. A myriad of new sauces, dishes, beverages and confectionary were created and fine-tuned, making French food irresistible to the human senses.

Gerome handed me my aromatic expresso and tiny almond biscuit, and with regret, added that while French cuisine is still in high demand worldwide, it is more and more difficult to find an authentic French restaurant, even in Paris.

At that moment, an elegant woman walked into the café, kissed 'hello' to Gerome, who then introduced her to me as Madame de Bonnières.

She was well-presented, in her mid-fifties with blond hair and natural make-up, which perfectly matched her open, talkative personality.

She was in charge of managing the kitchens of the most famous cabaret located nearby, and she was exactly the person I was looking for! After hearing me out, she smiled mysteriously and invited me to come to her restaurant at 7.30 pm.

It was mid-week, but the restaurant was packed with locals and tourists. Madame greeted me at the door and seated me at a small corner table covered with crispy white tablecloths, shiny cutlery, and empty glasses and plates.

The sommelier served champagne in traditional shallow champagne glasses called 'coupe', which allowed the bubbles to freely escape and tickle my nose. Seeing my delight, the hostess explained that the shape of the coupe was modelled on the breast of the French Queen Marie Antoinette, the wife of King Louis XVI of France. Since that moment, I have had a different perspective when it comes to champagne. It is no longer an alcoholic drink, but something which sets my mind in a certain frame – a thirst for sensual experience.

The 'le diner' menu was comprised of three pre-set six-course menus of either seafood, meat and vegetarian dishes with matching wine or non-alcoholic beverages. Everything on the menu looked delicious, and I was puzzled about which option would offer me the best chance to experience the aphrodisiac powers of French cuisine. Seeing my hesitation, and with an enigmatic smile, Madame confirmed that all three menus were equally charged with love-stimulating powers, and each would allow me to fully experience my introduction into the world of French orgasmic cooking ('cuisine orgasmique').

It was after eight pm and I was worried that the six-course dinner would be too much for me at that time of night, however I was assured that, according to the cannons of 'nouvelle cuisine', the accent is on quality, taste, originality and the presentation of the dishes, rather than on their quantity. Finally, I chose the seafood option.

After wishing me 'bon appetite', Madame went on with her duties as hostess of the establishment, while I was left to anticipate the discovery of mysterious French aphrodisiacs.

I looked around, noticing that every single detail had been carefully thought through and designed to discretely excite the different senses of diners and fire up their anticipation.

Crispy, white linen tablecloths contrasted with the cherry-coloured walls and upholstery on the comfortable chairs, even the shiny silver cutlery and monogrammed plates were discreetly escalating my expectations. The subtle, seductive music mixed with the soft voices of other diners provoked one's eyes to look around the room at other diners, and the air smelled of perfume mixed with the faint scent of musk and jasmine, which was obviously used strategically to relax, elevate mood and excite the emotions.

This atmosphere obviously worked, as while I sipped my aperitif, I noticed many total strangers trying to make eye contact with me, by locking eyes and bowing their heads. It was contagious and I soon found myself doing the same. To my surprise, this activity provoked in my mind certain romantic fantasies, which probably increased the level of phenylethylamine in my body, responsible for the feelings of romance, excitement and euphoria.

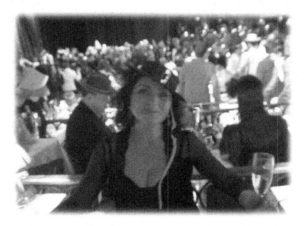

The hors d'oeuvre (appetiser) arrived while I was still sipping my champagne. It was a single freshly chucked natural oyster topped up with ossetra caviar and crème fraîche, which rested on a tiny plate full of sea salt. Madame came by my table and, pointing at the oyster with her well-groomed fingernail, said that while many knew about oysters' aphrodisiac magic, hardly anyone knew that the little topping of ossetra caviar, green watercress leaf and young cheese turned it into a love-bullet. She was right! The combination of the nutrients and certain essential fatty acids, vitamins and minerals, washed down with the taste-bud teasing action of the champagne, triggered feelings of arousal and anticipation. There is a certain affinity between oysters and eroticism, as our senses get excited by the sexy, luscious texture and pleasant sea-water smell, as well as the suggestive presentation of the shiny pink lustre of the shell and rich taste.

The second course was coquilles Saint-Jacques accompanied by small glass of chablis. It was made of fresh scallops, covered with hot creamy sauce and herbs, elegantly presented on the shells. To my surprise, this starter made me feel even hungrier than the previous dish. Once again it was loaded with fatty acids, which our body needs to produce hormones. Over the centuries, many world cuisines have included seafood on their menus as an effective aphrodisiac. Modern science has explained this phenomena by discovering high levels of essential fatty acids (those that cannot be synthesised by one's own body) in

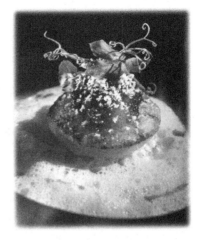

seafood, which feed, support and stimulate human sexuality.

The citrus notes of the sauce suggested that some citrus enzymes were involved in helping with digestion, while the flowery aromas of the white chablis perfectly cleansed my palate between morsels. My excited taste buds were screaming for more!

When the third course arrived I thought that I'd never eat it, as sardines are not my favourite fish. My wine glass was topped up with crispy chablis again, and out of respect to Madame, I decided to taste the sardines. Surprisingly, I could not stop eating them till my plate was totally clean. The combination of fresh-grilled sardines, topped with tangy, pungent herb-and-fennel crispy salad, stimulated my appetite and intensified the delicious feelings of arousal and eagerness. Once again I was left wishing that there was more of the dish on the plate, and was amazed with the response of my body and senses to the food. Perhaps my excitement was due to the wine, as alcohol is able to release inhibitions, and is known to act as an aphrodisiac when consumed with food in small quantities.

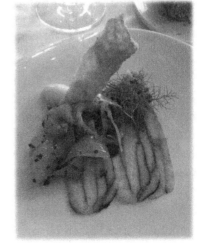

Busy with my thoughts and fascination with the whole experience, I didn't notice when the singer appeared on the little stage. Her mellow voice and sexy dress, combined with the light scent of musky perfume in the air and sensual music, perfectly blended into the soft light of the restaurant.

The fourth dish was lemon-scented lobster, pippies and black mussels served with ginger, caramelised chili and lemongrass, topped with light tomato-based sauce and edible lemon-scented herbs. The wine was from the Rhone Valley – Picpoul de Pinet – and it could be described as a match made in heaven! The green velvety sauce added a sexy feel to my mouth, which was teased by the chili and ginger. My over-excited taste buds made me feel sorry that there were only two more dishes left to try!

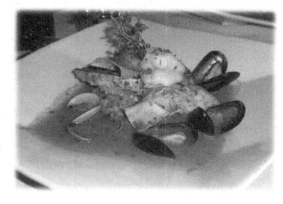

Analysing my feelings I realised that, once again, this clever recipe was playing with amino acids in different combinations with the greens and spices. This tasty, clever concoction subtly increased my neurotransmitter levels (norepinephrine and dopamine), which caused a sex-boosting effect.

With burning cheeks, I looked around and was amazed to see many silent guests totally absorbed in their feelings of pleasure under the spell of the soft music and tinkling cutlery. I realised that my physical and mental capacities were coming to the point of sweet orgasmic pain, and I shivered with ecstasy. I didn't want to eat anymore, but I didn't want to leave either!

The music became more alive with the rhythms of tango and chanson. Some couples were dancing, and that's when another piece of French magic was served. It was a porcelain spoon topped with a sherbet made from peppers, tomatoes, cucumbers and fresh herbs. Encouraged by the smiling Madame, I tried the cool, savoury sherbet with its crunchy texture and discovered that its refreshing flavour miraculously revitalised my taste buds and made me eagerly embrace the next dish.

Roasted turbot with a medley of fennel, leaks, potatoes (gratin dauphinois) and herbed chanterelle mushrooms came paired with a fine, dry white burgundy, which further cleansed my palate and added an interesting perspective to this highly aromatic dish.

I deliberately ate slowly, stretching out the unusual pleasure and wishing that it would never end. Some couples were kissing, others were speaking to each other only as lovers do. I wished that my husband was there.

How did this happen? I was stunned to realise that it was the combination of all the libido-enhancing components – the food, beverages, aromas, music, light and sensual atmosphere – that were working their powerful magic on the senses.

Fascinated with this discovery I could not wait to talk to Madame de Bonnières, and when she finally came to my table, I snowed her down with questions: Who was the mastermind that played so skilfully with human neurotransmitters and bodily functions? Who was behind the recipes with their delicately chosen elements that subtly directed the senses to such a delightful state of sexual arousal?

She smiled at my excitement which, without any words, proved that I had discovered the power of the famous French aphrodisiacs. She said that what I had experienced was the combined effort of her chefs, music director, interior decorator and coordinator, along with her interest in French culinary history, and, of course, she could not tell me the secret formulas of the food or the visual stimuli which they used. However, she assured me that everything I had experienced that night had been tested over a long time on millions of diners and what did not work was no longer used. I thanked her for the pleasant experience and congratulated her on an incredible achievement. Wishing me a pleasant rest of the night, Madame de Bonnières disappeared.

I don't like sweets, and hardly ever order desserts, however when the traditional French classic dish arrived – a dark chocolate soufflé with liquored white chocolate sauce – I unexpectedly had the urge to try it … and a few minutes later it was all gone. It was in perfect balance – light, not very sweet and sensually soft in the mouth. Once again, the tannins of the cleverly selected accompaniment (cabernet sauvignon from

Bordeaux) eased its digestion and sped up the process of its chemicals and elements in manipulating sensuality.

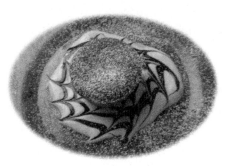

After that, I sipped my green tea deliberately slowly, frequently stopping to replay in my mind the whole experience and to watch the provocative cabaret show. The sexual elation bestowed on me by the end was obvious – it was overwhelming and I felt very sorry to be there by myself.

Remembering all the details of the dinner and its readily accessible ingredients, I still could not pinpoint exactly what had triggered those delicious, amorous feelings in me and what exactly gave French food its sex appeal.

Surprisingly, the six-course dinner did not leave me feeling too full. Perhaps because the courses were spaced out to almost three hours, or my calorie intake was just right for me.

I felt light, romantic, elated and sexually excited! But most of all I was happy with having discoved the secret to French aphrodisiacs – a perfect balance between food and other elements that stimulate the senses, all contributing to one common goal ... pleasure of sensual euphoria!

To Health, Long Life & Pleasures!

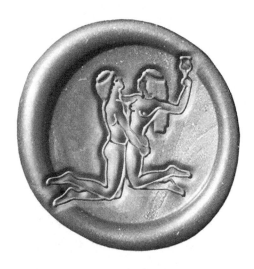

About The Author

Over thirty years ago Lillian Zeltser stumbled on an old love potion recipe, which sparked up her life-long interest to aphrodisiacs. Together with her husband, a medical doctor, she hunted for effective natural aphrodisiacs around the world, and was involved in many experimentations and extensive research.

In this book she shares some information about her discoveries, and some time-tested traditional recipes and captivating legends.

She lives in Melbourne (Australia) with her family and you can visit her online at AphrodisiacsExpert.com

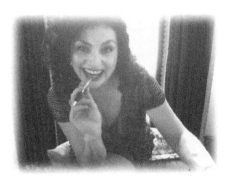

Made in the USA
Columbia, SC
21 December 2020